Contents at a Glance

Absolute Beginner's Guide

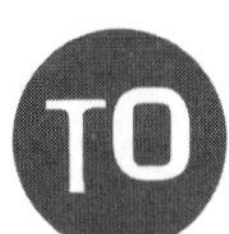

Pregnancy

John Adams, M.D. and Marta Justak

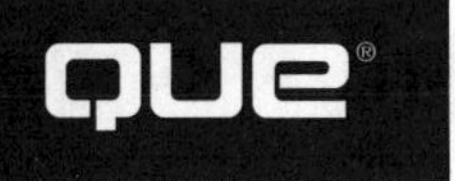

800 East 96th Street,
Indianapolis, Indiana 46240

Absolute Beginner's Guide to Pregnancy

International Standard Book Number: 0-7897-3216-5

Library of Congress Catalog Card Number: 2004107643

Printed in the United States of America

First Printing: October, 2004

07 06 05 04 4 3 2 1

Trademarks

All terms mentioned in this book that are known to be trademarks or service marks have been appropriately capitalized. Que Publishing cannot attest to the accuracy of this information. Use of a term in this book should not be regarded as affecting the validity of any trademark or service mark.

Warning and Disclaimer

Every effort has been made to make this book as complete and as accurate as possible, but no warranty or fitness is implied. The information provided is on an "as is" basis. The authors and the publisher shall have neither liability nor responsibility to any person or entity with respect to any loss or damages arising from the information contained in this book.

Bulk Sales

Que Publishing offers excellent discounts on this book when ordered in quantity for bulk purchases or special sales. For more information, please contact

U.S. Corporate and Government Sales
1-800-382-3419
corpsales@pearsontechgroup.com

For sales outside of the U.S., please contact

International Sales
international@pearsoned.com

Executive Editor
Candace Hall

Acquisitions Editor
Karen Whitehouse

Development Editor
Karen Whitehouse

Managing Editor
Charlotte Clapp

Project Editor
George Nedeff

Indexer
Mandie Frank

Proofreader
Carla Lewis

Publishing Coordinator
Cindy Teeters

Interior Designer
Anne Jones

Cover Designer
Dan Armstrong

Page Layout
Susan Geiselman

Graphics
Laura Robbins

Table of Contents

About the Authors

Dr. John Adams has been practicing medicine since 1993 when he received his Doctor of Medicine from Texas A&M University College of Medicine. Specializing in Obstetrics and Gynecology, he has served as a naval doctor in the U.S., Italy, and Iraq. Dr. Adams has personally delivered over 1,000 babies in his career and has dealt with any number of difficult and extreme medical situations. He is currently practicing in Denver, Colorado at Exempla Saint Joseph Hospital, where he is a member of the faculty teaching OB/GYN to residents and interns.

Marta Justak graduated from Duke University with a liberal arts degree, double-majoring in U.S. History and Comparative Area Studies (Far East and Latin America), which gave her a solid background for her future career in publishing. She's worked in all facets of the media, including television, radio, newspapers, magazines, and books, mostly as a writer and editor, but also as a publisher. For the past six years. Marta has focused on her own literary agency, Justak Literary Services, Inc., where she represents clients and packages books for publishers. But her greatest achievement is the fact that she's raised five children, of whom she is inordinately proud.

Dedications

To Kramer Justak, whose encouragement, thoughtfulness, and support I will never forget. You are truly an inspiration and helped me to turn this "idea" into a reality!

—John Adams, M.D.

To my parents, Ray and Martine Justak, who taught me how to love and inspired me to have my own family…and to my five children who gave the word "love" a new meaning.

—Marta Justak

Acknowledgments

Thank you Marta Justak. What fun this was! If I had known that co-authoring a book could be like this.... Talented and gifted individuals have been described as taking what must be a difficult and challenging task and making it look extremely easy to accomplish. You are such an individual! I could not have been more blessed to have had such a remarkable partner as you in this endeavor, and I have gained a special friend in the process.

My Family is such a big part of this book in so many ways. Always there for me providing love and support, they have inspired me to take chances and set high goals for myself. Thank you, Mom and Dad, for everything. To my beautiful sister, Janet, you are a constant and everlasting source of optimism and love for the whole Family that cannot be measured. Thank you to my brother-in-law Bill who "looks out" for me in so many different ways that I dare not mention here. And to my lovely nieces, Lisa and Laurie, who place me on a pedestal undeservedly so and make me so very proud of them.

I want to thank the U.S. Navy for helping me to "accelerate my life." The training I received was first class and the opportunities afforded me were, to say the very least, unforgettable. Most of all, it is the people who matter, and I will not forget those fine individuals who led by example as consummate professionals while at the same time managing to give something back to their country.

My sincere appreciation goes out to the leadership of Exempla Healthcare and Saint Joseph Hospital in Denver, Colorado, for their support and cooperation and for the use of some of the photographs in this book. Thank you to my colleagues Nick Peros M.D., Rachel Gaffney M.D., Chris Geising M.D., Jan Notch, Pascale Gomez, and Jim Smith M.D. Thanks to Barbara Hughes and the CNM staff as well as the support and encouragement of the clinical and nursing staff. I could not imagine a better group of colleagues to have the pleasure of working with. And a special thanks goes out to the Ob/Gyn Residents for allowing me the privilege to participate in your education and also for keeping me on my toes! You are the future indeed.

—John Adams, M.D.

In any book, you'll find a multitude of people behind the scenes, but there was one person up-front who had special meaning for me, and that would be my co-author, Dr. John Adams. Writing a book with a partner can run the gamut from being a breeze to a nightmare. In this case, John turned out to fit the former pattern, as he was an absolute joy to work with. John gave me unstintingly of his time night after night, and he never seemed to run out of patience as I pestered him with endless questions. In the process, I've come to think of John as a special friend. I shall miss having the excuse to chat with him every night, since our conversations often deviated from pregnancy onto philosophy, politics, music, and our all time favorite topic—anything related to the Mac and Apple products.

I'd also like to thank my sister, Kramer Justak, for introducing me to John. She and John worked together as part of the Navy medical support team at the front in Operation Iraqi Freedom. Kramer joined the Navy as a nurse after September 11, 2001. She is my own personal hero.

Special thanks to my parents who encouraged me to write and have always been there for me and my children in every way possible, to my sister, Nora, who has been a best friend as well as a loving sister, and to my own children, who keep my sense of humor intact with their antics (even though they should be beyond the "antic stage"). I have to say that my children represent the best creative work I've ever done. In fact, they did make pregnancy worthwhile!

Both John and I would like to thank the editorial and production team at Pearson for giving us the opportunity to write the book we wanted with minimal interference. Kudos and appreciation to Candy Hall for being a publisher with foresight.

Finally, we'd like to give a special salute and our undying gratitude to Karen Whitehouse, our editor on the project. I've known Karen for years and have worked with her in many capacities, but she never ceases to amaze me with her publishing wisdom and vision.

—Marta Justak

We Want to Hear from You!

As the reader of this book, you are our most important critic and commentator. We value your opinion and want to know what we're doing right, what we could do better, what areas you'd like to see us publish in, and any other words of wisdom you're willing to pass our way.

As an executive editor for Que Publishing, I welcome your comments. You can email or write me directly to let me know what you did or didn't like about this book—as well as what we can do to make our books better.

Please note that I cannot help you with technical problems related to the topic of this book. We do have a User Services group, however, where I will forward specific technical questions related to the book.

When you write, please be sure to include this book's title and author as well as your name, email address, and phone number. I will carefully review your comments and share them with the author and editors who worked on the book.

email: feedback@quepublishing.com

Mail: Candace Hall
Executive Editor
Que Publishing
800 East 96th Street
Indianapolis, IN 46240 USA

For more information about this book or another Que Publishing title, visit our Web site at `www.quepublishing.com`. Type the ISBN (excluding hyphens), or type in the title of a book in the Search field.

The Book Is a Baby (for Us)

Dr. John Adams (hereinafter referred to as *Dr. John*) and I met about a year ago through my sister. They were friends and co-workers in the Navy and served at the front in Iraq together. He and my sister (an OR nurse) along with their medical unit treated over 700 wounded U.S. soldiers (mostly Marines) and Iraqis in three weeks of war. To me, they are both heroes.

After serving in the Navy for 10 years, Dr. John left the military and now teaches OB/GYN residents and interns at a hospital in Denver, Colorado. He seemed like the perfect candidate to be a co-author to write this book, as he has personally delivered over 1,000 babies in his career and has dealt with any number of difficult and extreme medical situations.

OBS AT THE FRONT

Frankly, I always thought it was kind of nuts having an OB/GYN at the front. Let's face it—how many Marines are likely to come into the OR (operating room) who are pregnant or having a baby in the middle of a war? Dr. John laughingly agreed with me, but pointed out that his surgery skills qualified him to serve as an assisting surgeon. Hey, if you met him, you'd feel that he *was* capable of handling any medical emergency that came his way. And bottom-line: never argue with the U.S. Navy or Marines. Just go where they tell you.

So…I'm the writer of our team…and the mother who has had five children and six pregnancies (one miscarriage). When the publisher broached the idea of this book to me, I jumped at it and knew that I would call Dr. John to participate. We bring to this book a unique perspective—he's got the medical expertise, and I've been the unwitting patient five times over. I say "unwitting," because after writing this book I wish I could go back and do the pregnancies all over again. I never knew how much I didn't know! Oh, and I'm a writer, too, although I think having and raising five kids qualifies me a lot more.

How We Wrote This Book

We wrote this book as a team, albeit a separated one. John lives in Denver, and I live in Indianapolis. We spent many long hours on the phone with me interviewing John, asking endless questions, and him patiently explaining. Thank God for the Internet, as our chapters went winging back and forth at the touch of a button.

Because I literally "wrote" the book, the voice is more or less mine speaking; however, I often "speak" with the words that Dr. John gave me. Most of the snide asides are mine. (Dr. John's humor is droll, but not that droll.) Yet Dr. John patiently put up with my endless pleas to make things simpler and not go into too much detail, which I've decided is very difficult for a doctor to do. Trust me when I say that they always have a caveat for every situation. There were many times when I rolled my eyes and said, "We don't have to tell the reader every last thing," to which Dr. John would reply, "But we want to cover ourselves." (And for that orientation, we can give thanks to the insurance industry and lawyers!)

But I digress...

I wanted to work in stories from both of us, so you'll find sidebars entitled "From the Doctor's Perspective" and "From the Patient's Perspective." It was a gimmick that allowed us to deviate from the normal text and work in some amusing or personal events. Look for them and enjoy! You'll also find tips and notes and warnings (or cautions). Again, these devices are just additional ways to give you snippets of information in a more manageable fashion (translation: they are short).

There is an appendix of medical terms in the back. It is not complete, but certainly complete enough for you to grasp everything that we're discussing here. If you're truly lost or confused, try going online or better yet, discuss your questions with your doctor or healthcare professional.

Some of you may wonder why we didn't spend more time on midwives and their role in the birthing process. Although Dr. John has worked with midwives often and appreciates their expertise, we chose to focus on the doctor's role because that's where his expertise lies. We'll leave it to someone in the midwifery field to write that book. We did, however, give some information on their association and some advice on how and where to find a midwife.

HE VS. SHE

As an editor myself, I was often torn about the use of "he" versus "she" when referring to doctors, but it does make for an awkward sentence structure trying to cover your bases. Sometimes, I used "she," but more often I used "he," simply because it worked better so that the reader didn't confuse me and my voice with John's voice as the doctor. No slight was intended. My favorite OB (aside from John) was a female.

Why We Wrote This Book

We wrote it because we were asked to do so, of course. But beyond that, we wrote it because we felt we had something to say. I looked at other books that were out there, and there were definitely some good ones. But they didn't answer all my questions, and they weren't always user friendly, so to speak. We tried to fill in some of the gaps that the other books left open.

I love interviewing people so I think of endless questions. I finally had a captive audience in John (at least for a few hours every night), and I think you'll get some information that you've never heard before. For example, where else could you find the questions to ask a doctor from the doctor's perspective (see Chapter 2)? And who knew what was going on in a doctor's head while you were delivering (see Chapter 16)? Just reading all the things that happen from the doctor's viewpoint is fascinating.

And I have perspective from the mother's viewpoint and a sense of humor about pregnancy itself. When John would start pontificating about the "shoulds and should nots" of pregnancy, I'd pull him up short and tell him simply to "get a grip; no woman was going to be that perfect." Sometimes, however, I'd want to make light of a situation that he felt strongly about, so I'd compromise and let him have his way. In that way, we were a perfect team.

So, I hope you'll enjoy this book. I know we enjoyed the process of getting to know one another better and hopefully putting out a product that will educate women and help them take charge of their pregnancy in a positive way and have a wonderful relationship with whomever they choose as a healthcare professional. And remember—doctors are people, too!

PART I

PREPREGNANCY

In This Chapter

- Determining if you're pregnant
- Different kinds of pregnancy tests
- Emotional and physical symptoms of pregnancy
- How to tell the world your good news

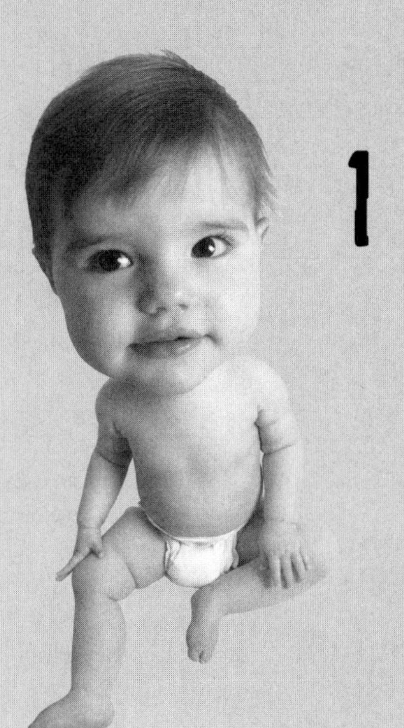

1

Finding Out You're Pregnant

The best of times…the worst of times…Finding out you're pregnant can be exhilarating, frightening, and downright baffling. You'll run the gamut of emotions from sheer joy to outright terror. It's not just the pregnancy you have to get through—it's all those emotions about becoming a parent.

After raising five kids, I can assure you that the parenting will take care of itself (believe it or not). Don't borrow trouble at this point. Focus instead on the pregnancy and how to make it a positive experience. After all, that's the only thing you can really marginally control at this point in time.

note

According to the National Center for Health Statistics (NCHS), there are over 4 million births in the U.S. each year

The Tests and Symptoms

First things first: Are you or aren't you pregnant? Most women find out they're pregnant by the tried and true method—that is, their period stops. So, if you miss a period, and you've been sexually active, it's safe to assume that you *could* be pregnant, and you *should* take a pregnancy test. You can either purchase a pregnancy kit at your local drugstore or go to a clinic (or your doctor) to have a test performed.

The Kits

Pregnancy kits come in all shapes and sizes (Figure 1.1). What they all have in common is that they are fairly easy to use. Basically, you urinate into a container and follow the instructions about what to do next. Usually, the test results occur in a matter of minutes. Sometimes, it's good to take a back-up test, particularly if you suspect the test is positive, but it turns up negative (called a false negative; there is also a false positive). A kit is not infallible; it can be wrong.

Personally, I panicked every time I took a pregnancy test—mostly because I freaked out that I would do something wrong (Figure 1.2). Sometimes, I coerced my husband into helping, but usually the directions were simple and easy to follow. There are even pictures if you really get confused. Sometimes, there are two tests in a kit, so if anything goes wrong, you have a backup.

FALSE NEGATIVE OR FALSE POSITIVE

Pay attention because this can get confusing. A false negative means that the pregnancy test indicated the test was negative (you aren't pregnant), but, in fact, it isn't really negative, it's really positive (you are pregnant). A false positive is the reverse (totally confusing, I know).

Any test that you can do on yourself has a false positive and a false negative rate. The manufacturers try to design a test to pick up the entire spectrum of possibilities from everyone who is normal to those who are abnormal. Unfortunately, making any test sensitive to everyone is impossible. For example, if you lower the test to pick up an abnormality, you may pick up a lot of false positives. When you design a test to rule out a problem (for example, you want it to come back negative in most instances), you will have a few false positives. Scientists try to minimize these instances, but they can't ever eliminate them, so they use a bell-shaped curve.

The upshot of this information for you is that if you know you're pregnant because your body is telling you something that the test doesn't, then repeat the test. Eventually, it should turn out positive; or preferably, have your doctor do the test. It's rare that the doctor will have a problem with the test, but it is possible.

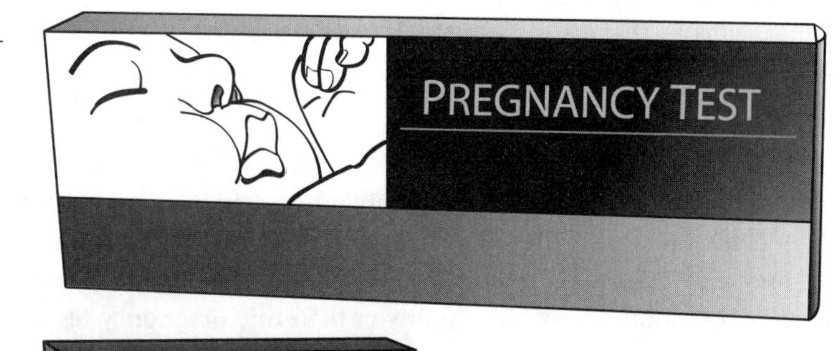

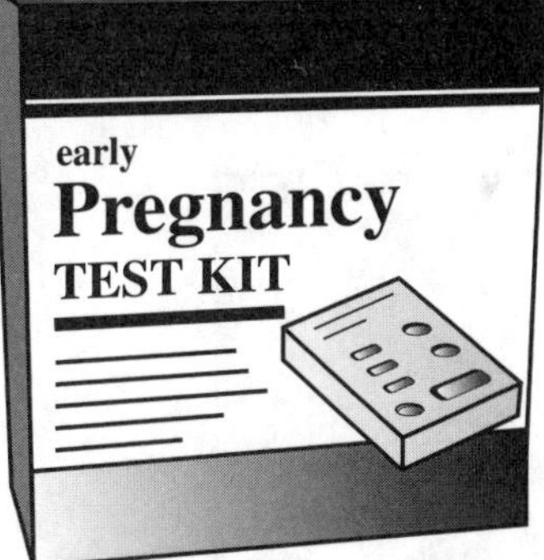

FIGURE 1.1
Pregnancy kits come in all shapes and sizes and are relatively inexpensive to purchase.

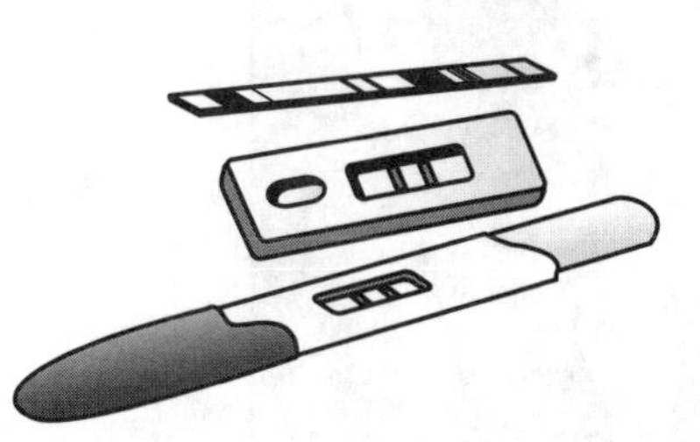

FIGURE 1.2
Pregnancy strips are color-coded and simple to interpret.

CASE HISTORY—NOTHING IS EVER 100% SURE

My friend Jane had been trying to get pregnant for years. Finally, she thought she was pregnant, but when the doctor gave her a pregnancy test (blood test) at his office that morning, it came back negative. As Jane continues the story, "I went home and within two hours of the doctor's test, I had a very strange bit of spotting or bleeding, but it didn't feel like a normal period. I'd heard that early in a pregnancy you could have some spotting that wasn't normal, so I took a home pregnancy test within a few hours of the doctor's test, and it came out positive. Obviously, I didn't believe the first test, so I took a second home pregnancy test a couple of hours later, and it was also positive. I called the doctor back because I was scheduled to have a D&C the next day. He said it was unlikely that I was pregnant because his test was probably more accurate than my home pregnancy test. Although the doctor still felt that I would need a D&C, he agreed to give me a repeat pregnancy test that afternoon anyway. The second test came out positive." Incidentally, Jane's son (the pregnancy that wasn't detected) is now 20 years old.

The Clinic

A test performed at a clinic is more reliable than a home pregnancy test (Figure 1.3). A lot of clinics do a urine test first simply because it's easier and cheaper, but sometimes they may elect to do a blood test for pregnancy. The blood test is usually done if there are questions about the validity of the urine pregnancy test or if the doctor needs to check a level of pregnancy hormone called a *Quantitative Beta HCG* (basically the exact level of pregnancy hormone in the bloodstream).

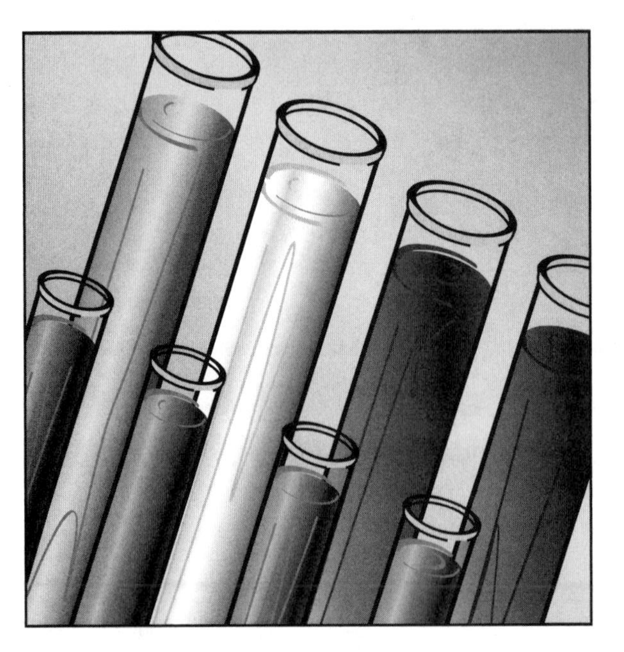

FIGURE 1.3
A blood or urine test taken in a laboratory is more reliable than a home pregnancy test.

A urine test and a simple blood test are examples of a qualitative test. In other words, these tests just indicate yes or no—either you're pregnant or you're not. A quantitative test measures the exact amount of hormones in the blood, which could help a doctor determine if the pregnancy is normal or abnormal. Typically, a doctor will order this test when he is worried about an *ectopic* pregnancy or a miscarriage.

note

An ectopic pregnancy is defined as an abnormal pregnancy located outside of the uterus. Usually, it leads to a miscarriage, and it can be dangerous and life-threatening to a patient. This is nothing to fool around with.

Watch out for that weight gain. Up to 20 weeks of pregnancy, the *average* weight gain is only 5–7 pounds, contrary to popular belief.

Physical and Emotional Symptoms

Some of the physical symptoms of beginning-stage pregnancy include breast tenderness, nausea, vomiting (morning sickness), feeling sick, tiredness, bloatedness, constipation and flatulence, and weight gain.

You may feel out-of-sorts emotionally and be a bit testier than usual with family and friends. (OK, you can be a hellcat on wheels, or cry without warning.) Things that normally wouldn't bother you may bother you enormously. You may feel depressed or have feelings of depression that are unexplained. Oddly enough, you may have an increased libido or sex drive and not know why. All of these symptoms can be attributed to pregnancy, so don't worry about them too much. They can also be attributed to an increase in hormones due to the pregnancy.

caution

However, if there is a possibility that you have depression for another reason—don't write it off. Or if your depression is severe, always, always seek professional help. Depression is not something to fool around with, and your physician can help you and *will* listen to you. If he or she doesn't listen and you're concerned, find a different doctor.

FROM THE MOTHER'S PERSPECTIVE...

I always knew that I was pregnant because I couldn't eat or drink some of my favorite foods and beverages without getting terribly queasy and sick to my stomach. For example, diet drinks made me ill, so my friends would always quip that I must be pregnant if I turned down a TAB (I know this dates me!). Sometimes, I also had a taste for different foods, particularly an increase in sugar (maybe not the best energy, but definitely quick). Hey, those pickle/ice cream stories in the middle of the night are true.

Cravings are a real function of pregnancy. I also remember wanting to sleep the entire first two months of my first pregnancy—a natural gestation period. I don't know when I've ever been so tired.

Telling the World

The best advice I ever received was to keep quiet about the pregnancy for as long as I was able (a difficult thing for me since I like to share with everyone). The reason is simple: miscarriages are fairly common. Approximately 20–30% of all pregnancies result in a miscarriage, which translates to one out of three pregnancies. Keeping those statistics in mind, you may want to wait to make sure your pregnancy is viable before telling the world. It's tough enough dealing with a miscarriage emotionally on your own without adding the sympathy and disappointment of family and friends. If you do think you're having a miscarriage, call your doctor immediately. You might need to have medical assistance.

Go ahead and make an appointment with your doctor when you discover that you're pregnant. Typically, doctors will schedule you for your first appointment when you're nine or ten weeks into your pregnancy. From that point on, you will probably see the doctor once a month until you reach 32–34 weeks at which point you will see the doctor every two weeks until you reach 37 weeks. After that, your appointments will likely be scheduled once a week.

FROM THE DOCTOR'S PERSPECTIVE...FIGURING OUT YOUR DUE DATE

As doctors, we determine the due date, or EDC (estimated date of confinement), calculated on approximately 40 weeks, beginning with the first day of the patient's last menstrual period. Doctors have a pregnancy wheel that calculates this fairly easily (Figure 1.4). They can also use computer programs. An easy way for a patient to figure out her due date is to use Naegele's Rule: take the first day of your last menstrual period, subtract three months, add seven days, and that should be your due date. We call it the poor man's OB calculator. Interestingly, it comes up to 40 weeks pretty consistently.

If you don't know when your last period was (perhaps because you were breast feeding, on birth control pills, or had an irregular menstrual cycle), then the best way to determine the baby's gestational age is to have an ultrasound.

Sometimes, patients ask us why we use their last menstrual period, rather than the date they thought they conceived or had sex. It's simple really. We've found that it's easier for a woman to remember her last menstrual period than to know when she last had sex. Plus, fertilization doesn't necessarily occur when the couple had sex.

The biggest "lie" of pregnancy is thinking that a baby's gestation is nine months. Actually, the average pregnancy lasts 40 weeks; if it were nine months that would translate to 36 weeks.

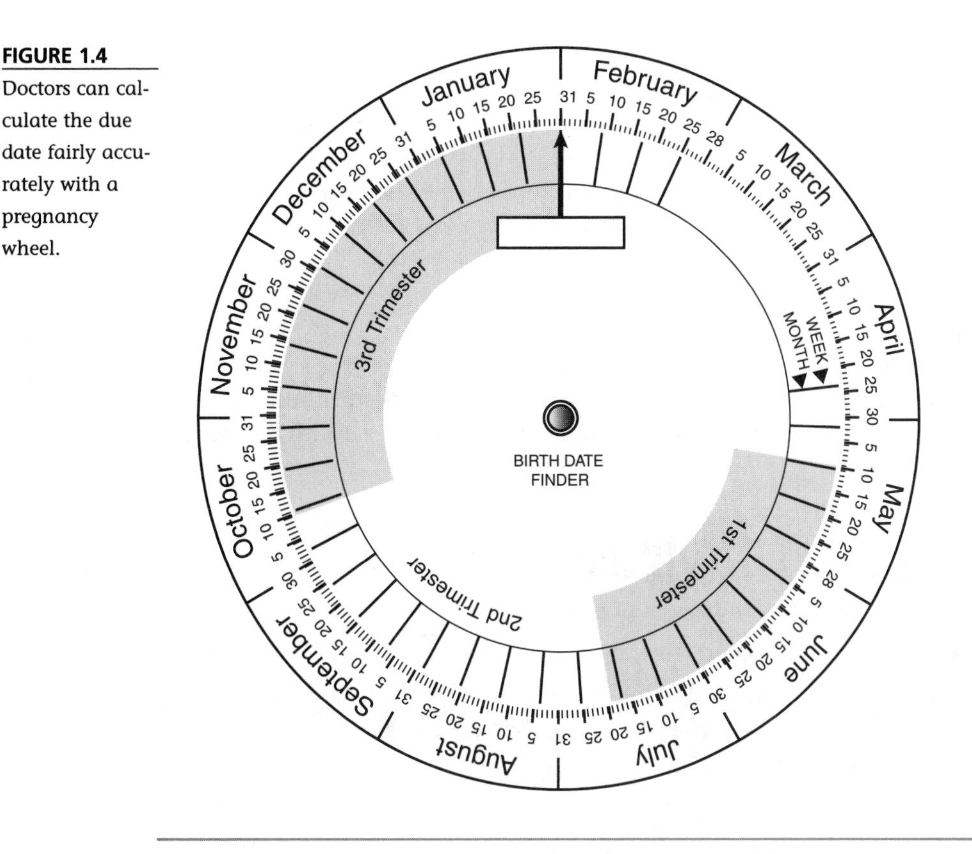

FIGURE 1.4
Doctors can calculate the due date fairly accurately with a pregnancy wheel.

Making Plans

OK, so you're pregnant. Where do you go from here? Sit down—take a deep breath—and "veg" for a bit. Squelch the urge to panic. Give into the excitement and joy. Scream if you need to. But above all, give yourself a chance to assimilate the news. You have plenty of time for planning—the baby won't be born for nine months or 40 weeks, give or take a few days or weeks. Right now—you, the mother, are the one who needs to be taken care of. If you feel like starting a list, here are some of the things you might put on it that are covered in subsequent chapters.

1. Choose a doctor (or midwife).
2. Choose a hospital.

3. Check insurance coverage (yours or your spouse's).
4. Check into maternity leave (if you're employed) or your spouse's paternity leave (if he has it).

DON'T GO HOG WILD JUST YET

Resist the urge to go on a spending spree, buying baby clothes, maternity clothes, diapers, cribs, and assorted baby paraphernalia. For one thing, people need something to give you for baby showers, so it's OK to look and make your lists at some retail stores, but it's too early to buy. For another, trust me on this one—you really don't want all that stuff sitting around staring you in the face for 10 months. It will make the time go even more slowly. You have almost a year to wait before the baby is born. Take it easy and don't rush something that can't be rushed—darn it, anyway!

Determining whether or not you are pregnant is the first task ahead of you. Once you've figured out that salient point, you can proceed with the rest of the book (and your life).

The Absolute Minimum

- First, find out if you're pregnant.
- Take a backup test if necessary.
- Make a list of the things you'll need to do—that is, finding a doctor, a hospital, checking your insurance coverage, and so on.
- Make a doctor's appointment.
- Shout your news from the rooftops.
- Get some sleep—you'll need it!

IN THIS CHAPTER

- The importance of choosing the right health care professional to deliver your baby
- The difference between an OB/GYN, a family practitioner, and a midwife
- Interviewing your doctor—some questions to ask
- Deciphering the answers, so they fit your needs

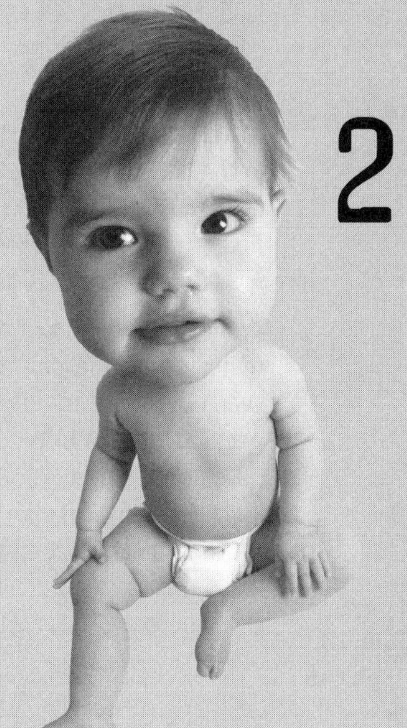

2

First Things First—Get Thee to a Doctor

Choosing a doctor is probably one of the most critical factors of your pregnancy, but if you're like me, it's not an area that you want to address. It just feels too hard trying to figure out where to find a doctor and which one matches you. If you already have an OB/GYN, you're the lucky one. If not, just how do you choose the doctor who is right for you?

MATERNAL MORTALITY RATE

In the U.S., the national maternal mortality rate is approximately 8–10 per 100,000 live births. *Note: This figure is approximately six to eight times less than it was in 1960 (see Figure 2.1).*

Worldwide mortality, however, equals approximately one maternal death every minute of every hour, 365 days a year, which in a comparative ratio equals 550 women per 100,000 live births. Women in the U.S. and Europe have about a 1 in 1,000 lifetime chance of a pregnancy-related death; whereas women in areas of African have a 1 in 25 chance of an obstetric-related death.

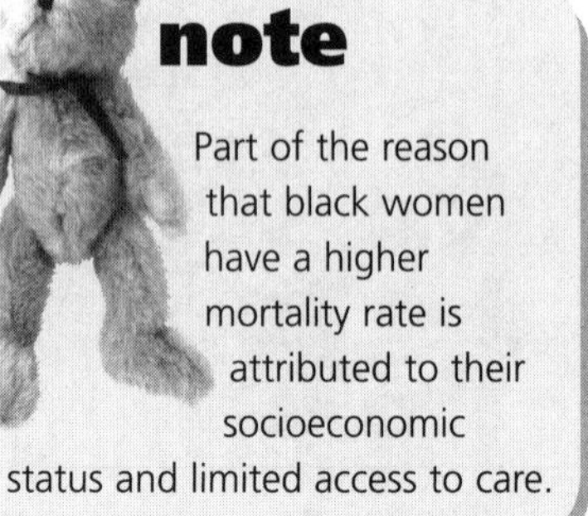

note

Part of the reason that black women have a higher mortality rate is attributed to their socioeconomic status and limited access to care.

FIGURE 2.1

As the chart indicates, the total maternal mortality rate in the U.S. over a 10-year period is less than 10 per 100,000 live births. Unfortunately, the rate among black women is still higher.

Maternal Mortality Rates

Maternal deaths per 100,000 live births

25
20
15
10
5
0

Black

Total

Year 2000 targets

1987 1990 1992 1994 1997 2000

Maternal deaths are those assigned to ICD-9 630-676 Data for 1997 are preliminary

Actually Finding a Doctor

There are many ways to find a doctor, but probably the best way is through word-of-mouth. Talk to your friends who have had babies and get recommendations from them. Did they like their doctor, was he or she easy or difficult to talk to, what are his/her credentials? However, remember that the same doctor who suits your friend may not be a match for you.

FROM THE DOCTOR'S PERSPECTIVE...

When I was in Jacksonville, Florida in the Navy making rounds, an intern once looked at me quizzically and said, "Can I ask you something?" I replied in the affirmative. "You know," he said somewhat smugly, "We're all doctors here. Isn't this pregnancy stuff a little overblown? Women have been having babies since the beginning of time. They had them at home, not in the hospital. Are we doing this all for the benefit of doctors, the hospital, and the insurance companies?"

I was stunned. I couldn't believe that a physician was asking this question. So I replied, "I'm going to give you some statistics, and we'll think about this question you asked. Since the turn of the century, the number of deaths attributed to pregnancy has dropped and the number of babies surviving has increased. Maternal mortality and infant mortality have fallen drastically in the last century. Fewer than 5 women per 100,000 will die of a pregnancy-related complication. Contrast that with the past when the number of women who died was in the range of 10–20 per 1,000.

"The top three causes of maternal death are amniotic fluid embolism, complications from pre-eclampsia, and hemorrhage. Are any of these top three causes something you could treat at home?" He shook his head, acknowledging that he could not.

I continued. "People expect perfection from doctors, and it comes as a complete shock to people these days when a woman dies in pregnancy because it's such a rare occurrence. But pregnancy can still be a life-threatening condition. In the time it takes for a woman to get from her home to the hospital, she could die."

Dr. John rested his case (see Figure 2.2).

Marta's note: Dr. John sounds a lot like Dr. *Phil. No wonder—they're both from Texas. At least he didn't say, "That dog won't hunt."*

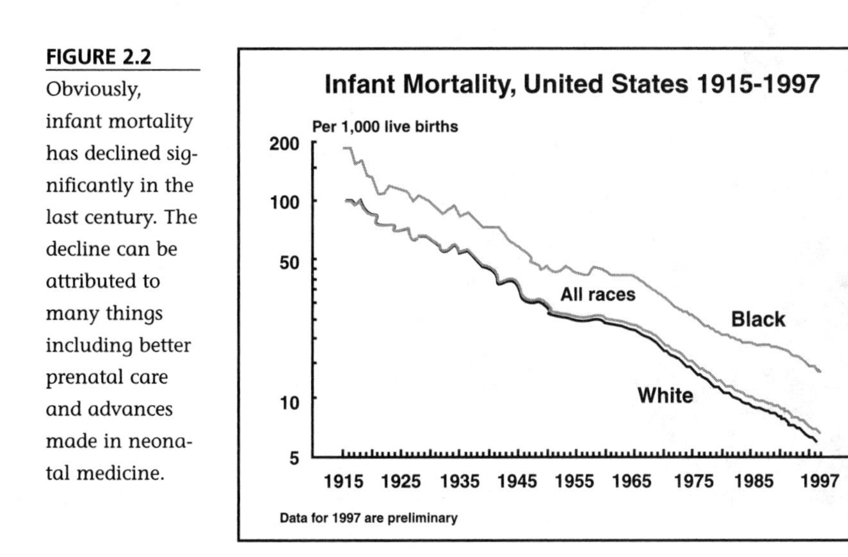

FIGURE 2.2
Obviously, infant mortality has declined significantly in the last century. The decline can be attributed to many things including better prenatal care and advances made in neonatal medicine.

Next question: Do you want an OB/GYN (obstetrics/gynecology) or a family practitioner? Both are physicians, but their areas of interest are vastly different.

> **note**
>
> A family practice physician studies for three years as a resident, focusing on a wide variety of medical disciplines.
>
> ---
>
> An OB/GYN completes a four-year residency, focusing only on women's health, primarily obstetrics and gynecology.

Family practitioners are primary care physicians, which means they take care of a wide range of medical problems or conditions that their patients may face. Their patients run the gamut of all ages—from babies through geriatrics. Family practitioners have a breadth of knowledge on most disciplines of medicine, and many of them will manage and deliver generally uncomplicated pregnancies. However, a family practitioner is also trained to know when to consult a specialist, such as an OB. If a pregnancy or labor gets to a point where there are complications, generally a family practitioner will consult an OB for advice, and the OB might assume the care of the patient.

The OB/GYN (see Figure 2.3) specializes in women's health and obstetric issues, both low- and high-risk cases. Typically, the OB/GYN will have a significant amount of experience in managing pregnancies and delivering babies, for obvious reasons—that's all the OB focuses on—pregnancy and women's health concerns.

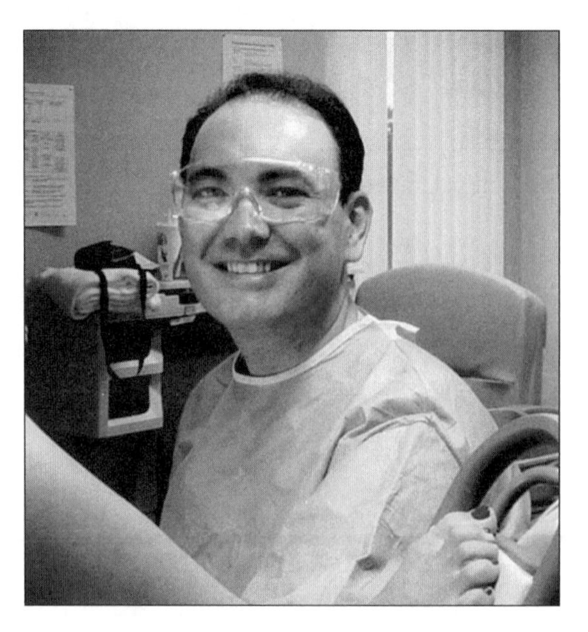

FIGURE 2.3
Here is a picture of Dr. John Adams (a certified OB/GYN) practicing his profession.

FROM THE DOCTOR'S PERSPECTIVE

OB/GYNs and FPs (Family Practitioners), as well as Certified Nurse Midwives (CNMs), are colleagues of one another—each with their respective roles and areas of expertise in caring for pregnant women. One of our jobs as an OB is to act as a consultant for FPs and CNMs. We're happy to assist as necessary, but always encourage them to call us as soon as possible if a patient has problems. If the OB is consulted sooner rather than later, then potential problems might be avoided.

Hospitals will give you lists of their doctors, but even better, go to the hospital of your choice and talk to nurses. Nurses always know who the best doctors are. You can check with a hospital to see if they will provide a doctor's credentials and ask if there is any litigation pending against that doctor, but hospitals are not necessarily required to divulge that information.

You can check with your state board of medical examiners to find out if the doctor you've selected has had many complaints filed against him/her. Doctors get on that list when a hospital is compelled to report them. If a hospital deems that a physician has committed an unwarranted act or poses a danger to patients, the hospital can and will suspend a physician's privileges until an investigation is completed. Hospitals don't want to be sued, therefore usually they won't hesitate to suspend a physician if they feel it is justified. However, suspension is a very serious offense, which could adversely affect a physician's career so hospitals will only proceed with this course of action if they deem it necessary.

caution

Keep in mind that some of the statistics you might find may be unfair and not reflect the truth of the matter because sometimes numbers don't tell you everything. Lawsuits can be filed that go nowhere (unsubstantiated) and are frivolous in nature, but they are still on record. Also, in today's litigious society, a good doctor may have cases that were settled by the insurance company, but the doctor was not necessarily found to be at fault. The insurance company simply deemed it cheaper and easier to settle.

Midwives

Some women may prefer someone other than a physician to care for them. Certified Nurse Midwives (CNMs) are an acceptable alternative to physicians. Rest assured that the majority of nurse midwives consult with OB/GYNs for any particular patient concerns they may have, but they act autonomously for most uncomplicated pregnancies. Although some midwives will perform a "home delivery," the majority of them prefer to deliver babies in a hospital setting where there are obvious advantages. In addition, midwives may offer a different "flavor" of care; for example, alternative ways to address pain or manage labor. Plus, the high likelihood of having a female midwife (although there are a few men) appeals to many women.

There are two types of midwives: those who are certified nurse-midwives and those who are not nurses but are still certified. The key word is *certified.* Make sure your midwife is certified if that's the way you choose to go. Here are two definitions of both certification types, taken from the Web site *www.midwife.org*.

- **Certified Nurse Midwives** are registered nurses who have graduated from a nurse-midwifery education program accredited by the American College of Nurse-Midwives (ACNM) Division of Accreditation (DOA) and have passed a national certification examination to receive the professional designation of certified nurse-midwife. Nurse-midwives have been practicing in the U.S. since the 1920s.
- **Certified Midwives** are individuals who have or receive a background in a health-related field other than nursing and graduate from a midwifery education program accredited by the ACNM DOA. Graduates of an ACNM accredited midwifery education program take the same national certification examination as CNMs but receive the professional designation of certified midwife.

caution

There are many people out there who say they are capable of taking care of pregnant women or claim some level of authority or expertise, but they have no formal training or education. These individuals should be avoided, as they have no legal accountability or responsibility for the patient's ultimate welfare.

note

If the patient desires a coach or a *doula*, this is acceptable as long as that person is not your primary caretaker. *Remember: Take the doctor's advice over the coach or doula.* Sometimes, it becomes a competition between the doctor and the coach as to who is "right." This is an unhealthy situation for the patient.

A Counseling Session with a Doctor

Here is a little known fact about doctors. They really wish that you would get in to see them and counsel with them *before* you get pregnant, rather than *after*. That way they can react to a medical problem you might have *before* the pregnancy, rather than *afterwards* when it might be too late. It's particularly important with women who might have medical considerations factoring into their pregnancy. At this point, the doctor could tell you what your options for pregnancy are and whether or not you're a high-risk patient. Factors that might be important to discuss with your doctor ahead of time are:

- Current health and past medical history
- Age of mother
- Heart and/or lung problems
- Drinking or smoking
- Past pregnancy-related history

Another little known fact about doctors: they take what some patients say with a grain of salt (and I thought they believed everything we told them).

THE DOCTOR'S PERSPECTIVE...

Most of the time when we query a patient, we know that whatever they're telling us, it may not be the entire truth. For example, a patient will underestimate by three or four the number of cigarettes she smokes per day. We can tell a woman what we think she should do, but we realize that she will end up doing what she wants to do when we're not around. Fortunately, most people want to do the right thing. As doctors, we do, however, document everything we tell a patient—for our own protection as well as theirs. The record needs to be complete so that everyone knows the patient's correct history (as closely as possible) when the woman is in labor.

Interviewing Your Doctor

Don't be afraid to do background research about potential doctors ahead of time. If you have any friends who have had babies, ask them about their doctors. The best way to find a doctor is usually by word-of-mouth. I went through three different doctors (and three babies) before I found the doctor who was right for me (for the last two babies). I wouldn't suggest that route. It was nicer to have the same doctor for several babies—at that point I felt as if the doctor and I were friends, and she had a vested interest in me.

Another factor to consider is whether or not you're more comfortable with a man or a woman. I've had both—three babies with three different male doctors; two with the same female doctor. If you get an empathetic man (like Dr. John, of course), a male doctor is just fine; however, I found the female doctor to be more in tune with me (plus her hands were smaller—those exams, you know). The important part is that all of my doctors were there when I needed them and were highly competent physicians.

Remember, you're not just interviewing the doctor, but also his staff. Pay attention to the details. Do the nurses and assistants seem friendly and concerned? Do they answer your questions? How long is your stay in the waiting room?

POINT-COUNTERPOINT... "THE PATIENT'S"

OK, I admit that I once walked out of a waiting room after waiting for over two hours for my first appointment with a new doctor. Hey, I think my time is as valuable as the doctor's time. While I appreciate that doctors may have emergencies, I thought the staff should either have rescheduled me or gotten me in to see someone else. I crossed that doctor off my list and made an appointment with someone else.

POINT-COUNTERPOINT... "THE DOCTOR'S"

It's hard to tell why the doctor is running late if you haven't been seen in an appropriate amount of time. Some situations are unavoidable, but that doesn't excuse the fact that the staff should keep you informed of how long your wait will be, have you see another provider if available, or reschedule you for another visit. However, sometimes there are emergencies that the doctor must attend to, or the patients ahead of you may be taking more of the doctor's time than he or she had planned. Unfortunately, this happens a lot. On the other hand, most doctors will try to give you the same amount of care and attention as needed.

What Questions Should I Ask?

Here we list some questions to ask the doctor when interviewing him, and then give you how the doctor should (or should not) answer the questions.

After Dr. John responds (in italics) how he would answer the question with his patients, then he tells you what you should look for in the responses of your doctors.

1. How long have you been delivering babies?

My response is that I have been delivering babies for over 10 years.

However, there is no magic number here. Obviously, a doctor who has been practicing three years will probably have fewer babies delivered than one who has practiced 20 years. But again, that is not always the case. For example, you may have a doctor who only delivers a few babies a year vs. one who delivers all the time. On the positive side, the doctor who has only delivered a few will probably spend more time with you. On the negative side, he probably hasn't seen as many complications as a doctor who delivers more frequently. This is a subjective answer, depending on what you're looking for. My suggestion is that you look for someone who has the experience that you're comfortable with as a patient. You want to make sure that the doctor you're entrusting your pregnancy to has the right amount of experience to handle your case.

2. How many babies have you delivered?

Personally, I have delivered over 800 babies, but I worked at a military hospital where I saw a lot of patients.

Also, keep in mind that while a new doctor may not have delivered as many babies in her practice, she may have delivered quite a few as a resident. Again, this answer is similar to the one above. Not an exact number, but someone who has delivered 100 babies or more probably has some experience, rather than someone who has delivered fewer than 10. What is your comfort zone, i.e., the answer that gives you comfort? It's subjective and differs from one patient to another. Basically, what you want is a doctor who has had some experience and can handle problems with confidence and competence.

3. Do you have a preference for obstetrics or gynecology?

In my case, I like both—I like a balance. I like taking care of pregnant women and delivering babies, and I also enjoy women's health care in general.

Usually, OB/GYNs do have their preferences. Often, a doctor will decide to just pursue gynecological patients after a stint at delivery. Delivering babies at all hours does impede on a doctor's home life, so there is a high burnout rate. Also, if a doctor chooses a specialty such as high-risk OB, she probably likes it more.

Obviously, some OB/GYNs have a good balance in their practice and enjoy covering both areas. But there are some doctors who would rather do more gynecology than obstetrics. Asking the question, depending on the answer you receive, may let you know if the doctor is someone you want to follow your pregnancy. Another good reason is that if you want to have more children and you find out that your doctor is getting out of delivery soon, you might want to start with another doctor who will last through all your pregnancies.

4. What percentage of your deliveries is C-section?

My percentage of C-sections is probably around 18%.

This question should be answered with a percentage figure because you will probably *not* get exact numbers. In the U. S. we are seeing an increasing trend for babies to be delivered by C-section. That figure will probably get higher. Currently, the average number of C-sections is 22 24% in the U.S.

If your doctor quotes a higher percentage for C-sections or complications, it may *not* mean that he has a preference for doing that surgery, but rather that he has more high-risk patients. However, if your doctor follows relatively uncomplicated patients in his practice and has a higher percentage rate than the national average, you might want to follow up your question with "why."

What you want to find out is if your doctor is going to recommend a C-section for you in circumstances that are equal with another doctor who might choose to do a vaginal delivery. In general, C-sections carry more risk for the patient and baby; however, there are times when it is necessary and the risks of a C-section are outweighed by the risks of a vaginal delivery.

5. What is your complication rate?

This is a good question. My complication rate is low. I'm very pleased with that. I think I'm very fortunate, but I'm also well trained. I have very few problems or outcomes associated with the patients I manage. I also realize that complications are a fact of practicing medicine.

The real question here is whether or not your doctor will be honest with you. You won't know until you ask, although frankly, this question may take him/her by surprise. If the doctor gets defensive, is evasive, or offended, you may think twice about using that particular doctor. If the doctor is confident in his abilities, he will probably tell you. Most patients don't ask their doctors this question, so I'm sure I'll get some mail from doctors asking what in the heck I was thinking of...

What we're talking about is what percentage of deliveries is associated with problems as a result of the doctor's management of the patient. Granted, doctors have big egos, so they won't admit this very often. But hospitals do track internally the statistics on complications and doctors' names are attached to these cases, although hospitals don't advertise these numbers. Any doctor will have complications—it could be anything from something that happened in surgery to a readmission to the hospital from infection after a pregnancy. And some outcomes that are considered complications are unavoidable. Remember that the vast majority of doctors do want to take care of their patients.

6. What are your feelings about doing episiotomies?

I only do episiotomies if they are clinically indicated. I do not routinely do them, nor do I shy away from ever doing them. If a situation arises where I deem it necessary to improve the patient's delivery outcome, I would not hesitate to do one. However, I don't think they should be routine, although some doctors claim they have really good outcomes with them.

Some doctors routinely do episiotomies because they figure that a natural tear (if you let it tear naturally) can be more difficult to repair than a deliberate episiotomy. That can be true; however, a woman doesn't always tear. A doctor may also decide to cut if the woman is already starting to tear, or if it looks like it would improve the delivery of the baby.

7. How do you handle pain medication during the delivery? How early do you offer it?

I think it's important that the patient be as comfortable as possible, so I do offer medications to relieve discomfort during the labor and delivery process. I would discuss it in advance with my patient and respect her opinion if she wanted to have a natural birth without pain medications. If she changed her mind, I would offer her something.

Keep in mind that there are risks involved in taking pain meds and timing is important as well. For example, giving an epidural too early has been linked with an increased C-section rate because studies suggest that the epidural slows down labor. The medicine can slow down labor to the point where it doesn't allow further dilation of the cervix, so a C-section results.

The OB determines when you should get the pain medicine, not the anesthesiologist, who is basically a consultant. Doctors rarely will say that a patient can't get pain meds unless there is a medical contraindication for giving them. On the positive side, a patient who is comfortable with pain medication will likely increase her chances of having a successful vaginal delivery. There are some women who don't want any pain medication, and we should respect that choice. If a doctor says he'll always give it, that woman might not like that response and should choose a different doctor.

BEWARE

- Of a doctor who is inflexible about meds.
- Of a doctor who doesn't offer any meds.
- Of a doctor who overuses pain medicine (there are risks to fetus and mother in this case).
- Of a doctor who says you won't have any pain at all (giving too many meds or giving them too early can harm the patient or the baby).

---

8. Will you personally be delivering my baby or another doctor? Who is your backup?

I will do my very best to be the doctor who will deliver your baby; however, it is possible I may not be available on the very day you go into labor. If that situation does arrive, then a close associate of mine would be asked to deliver you and manage your labor and delivery. And I would introduce you to various providers in my group who might deliver you.

The doctor should know her vacation schedule and more or less whether or not she will be out of town around the time of your delivery. All doctors have backups. You need to know who the backup is and have a name to call if necessary, although the hospital should also have the backup name on file for your doctor and will also place the call.

9. Will my charts be available if you're not the doctor?

Yes—the short answer.

If you were to deliver at a different hospital than planned, your records would be sent over or faxed from the hospital you'd chosen. If the delivery is after hours, there is someone who may have access to the doctor's records. Some hospitals still use paper documentation, but increasingly, more hospitals use electronic documentation, so they will have immediate access to files.

10. When should I call you if I have a problem and what type of problem would necessitate a call?

Whenever you have a concern that you're not sure about, then that's good enough for me. Call and ask because you may have a serious question or problem. If you're unsure, then call anyway. It's better to be safe.

At times, symptoms may be considered minor, yet at the same time, they may provoke anxiety or concern in the patient about how well the pregnancy is going. If a patient is concerned, she should not hesitate to call her doctor. At other times, symptoms may be more obvious, for example, vaginal bleeding or unusual pain that is not improving or any type of leakage that could indicate her bag of water might have broken. At this point, there would be concerns about infection. Or perhaps the baby hasn't moved when the mother knows it should. These are all examples of problems that should be addressed immediately.

The Absolute Minimum

Choosing the *right* health care professional is probably the most important decision of your pregnancy, the key word being "right," which means someone who suits your personality and needs.

- Investigate your options with regard to health care professionals. Decide what you want and then go after it. If necessary, make a list of important criteria that you want in a doctor/midwife.
- Don't be afraid to interview the doctor or midwife whom you are thinking about choosing to deliver your baby. Treat them with respect, but ask difficult questions. You are the customer. You have a right to be choosy.
- If your gut intuition tells you that this health care professional isn't right for you, thank them and move on. Don't worry about hurting someone's feelings. Chances are good that the doctor/midwife you choose wants to be as comfortable with you as you are with them.

In This Chapter

- Should I look for the doctor first or the hospital?
- Questions to ask the hospital when you visit.
- Important criteria that your hospital should fulfill.
- Extras that might appeal to your fancy.

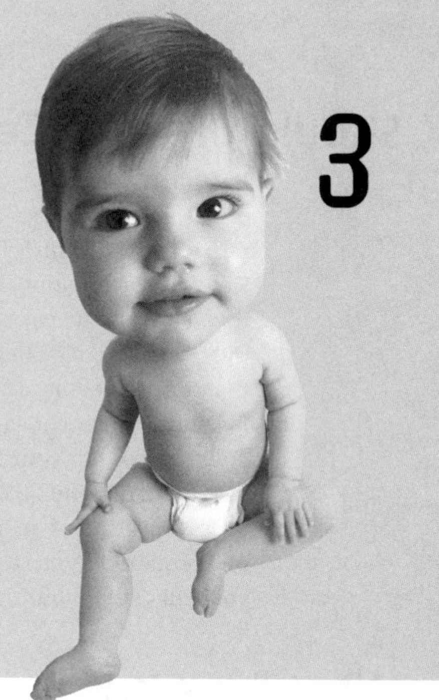

3

Choosing the Right Hospital

Many women have never been a patient in a hospital before the birth of their first baby, so they have absolutely no idea what to expect. The idea of even going to a hospital as a patient can be daunting. Fortunately, today's hospitals try to make the experience as "painless" as possible by offering all the comforts of home, and then some.

Should the Cart Come before the Horse?

If you have insurance (and here's hoping you do), then you may not have a choice of hospitals. Chances are good that you are limited by a specific list of preferred providers as to which hospital and health care provider (i.e., doctor) you can choose. However, being limited doesn't necessarily mean that you *don't* have a choice. Even if you have only two hospitals to choose from, go visit them in advance to see what they have to offer. Sometimes, women fall in love with a particular hospital that their doctor doesn't deliver in, and they choose to switch doctors in order to go to the hospital of their choice. You are the consumer here. Make sure that you get what you want within your means. If you have multiple choices for your hospital, then visit them all. The differences might be subtle, but you should still make the decision as to what kind of environment makes you comfortable. And even if you only have one hospital in your area, thus negating a choice, you should still visit to see what you will get for your money.

What Makes Hospitals Different from One Another

The choices are endless in today's hospitals as they compete for your dollars in the marketplace. Here is what one local hospital in my area (St. Vincent Women's Hospital in Indianapolis) offered on their Web site, touting how they were different from all the others (I've put my comments in parentheses):

- Free parking (This feature is always a good thing; parking can get expensive for your family and friends who visit.)
- Easy in and out for services and visiting (I think this means that it's easy for people to visit you—sometimes a good thing, but not always.)
- Conveniently located near the interstate (It depends on where you're coming from whether or not this matters to you; however, it might be convenient for your visitors. Of course, if you're in labor, you want the hospital that is closest to your location and to heck with everyone else's needs.)
- 24-hour room service meals at your request (I would have killed for this because after you deliver, you will be very, very hungry, and in the "old" days, you simply had to wait for the regular meals at regular times. This sole concept would move the hospital to the head of the list in my book, but then "hotel service" when you're in a hospital sounds simply decadent and wonderful to me.)
- Complimentary massages (A "to-die-for" idea, even if they only last 15 minutes—you can schedule them for longer and pay for them.)

- Free daily newspaper (Who has time to read or wants to waste time on a newspaper after having a baby—a negligible service in my estimation, although one the father might like.)
- Exclusive new baby portrait photography is available at your option (Most hospitals have some kind of photography service; in the past, the nurses took the pictures. The difference at this hospital is that you have a professional photographer available who will do unusual shots, rather than the standard ones—of course, expect to pay more.)
- All private rooms for obstetrical patients (I like this idea as well. I shared a room once—and only once—because it was an abysmal experience since my roommate cried the whole time because her baby was jaundiced.)

In addition, in-depth brochures from the same hospital highlighted their level IV neonatal unit, their extensive childbirth classes, and a new mother's support group that women can attend after their baby is born. This hospital offered tours twice a month for parents to attend and get the lay of the land. In fact, most hospitals today have similar programs.

BIRTHING OPTIONS

I remember once upon a time when it was in vogue to deliver a baby in a birthing pool under water. I'm not sure what the latest birthing options are, but if you want something out of the ordinary, make your requests known early and make sure that the hospital and your doctor will accommodate your requests, assuming they aren't too kinky.

So What Should Be Important to You

The most important thing is for you to feel comfortable with the staff and the environment of the hospital that you choose. Are the people friendly? Do you have confidence in their abilities? Some hospitals offer LDRP rooms, which translates to Labor Delivery Recovery Postpartum, meaning that you will be in the same room where you delivered until you go home. Other hospitals have a labor and delivery room, but then move you to a regular room on the maternity floor after you deliver. Do you want a private room (who doesn't want one?) or a semi-private room? Does the hospital even offer semi-private rooms at reduced costs? Previously, maternity rooms looked like any other hospital rooms. Today's maternity rooms often have carpeting and look more like luxury hotel rooms than anything remotely affiliated with a hospital. For example, all the oxygen outlets are hidden behind wooden cabinets. In fact, in some hospitals, the baby warmer in the mother's room folds down from the wall like an old-fashioned ironing board. There is a lot of effort that goes into designing labor and delivery rooms these days. Many hospitals, in an effort to compete, will go to great extent to offer the most positive experience when you have your baby.

> **tip**
>
> Many hospitals offer online enrollment for their childbirth classes. Check the hospital's Web site and search for classes that fit your schedule. (You might also find some classes on Lamaze, classes for prospective fathers or siblings, etc.) Often, these classes are offered for free, but you do need to enroll in advance of the class.

The first step is to call the hospital and schedule an appointment or time to visit. Go in armed with a list of questions, like you had for your doctor. Here are some questions that you might pose:

- What are the hospital's visiting hours for family and friends? Can they visit all the time or are there restrictions?
- Will I have one nurse assigned to me or will she take care of other patients at the same time?
- Do you have doctors on-call in case my doctor doesn't make it to the delivery room in time? Are these doctors residents or fully-fledged staff members?
- What would the normal procedures be if my pregnancy developed complications?
- What is the extent of your neonatal care? What level of neonatal care do you offer? If something goes wrong with the birth, would you send the baby to another hospital in the area? Which hospital?
- Are we allowed to take pictures during the birth process?
- Can my spouse or significant other be present during a c-section if I have to have one?
- How many people can be present in the delivery room?
- What kind of delivery rooms do you have?
- What "extras" does your hospital offer?
- How would you characterize the difference between your hospital and other hospitals?
- Are all of your rooms private or are some semi-private?
- Is there any way to cut costs if I'm paying for it myself—that is, I don't have insurance?
- Do you have a stocked refrigerator on the unit for patients who are hungry or deliver after hours, or do you offer room service at all times?

- Can my husband or significant other stay with me the entire time? Is there a bed or a couch for that person?
- What are the procedures for checking out and in? Are they lengthy or do you handle them in advance?
- Do you have free parking? If not, what are the charges?
- What kind of childbirth classes do you offer?
- Do you have a person on staff to teach new mothers how to nurse?
- What kind of follow-up care is available after the patient is released? Do you have a support nurse who can answer questions?

tip

Find some women who have had babies recently and ask them about their experiences with their doctors and their hospitals. New mothers love to talk about their labor and delivery "adventure." Find out what happened to them and what they did and didn't like about their hospital and/or doctor. Keep in mind that different people like different things and have different tastes. Still, at this point, you're simply collecting information. You can make a decision when you have all the information in place.

These are some of the questions you might ask. If you think of any others, jot them down on a list. In all likelihood, many of these questions will be answered on your tour before you even ask them.

While you're taking your tour, look around at the facilities. Is everything neat and clean? Cleanliness is of paramount concern in a hospital where bacteria and germs are at a premium. You want to minimize yours and your baby's risk for getting an infection.

FROM THE MOTHER'S PERSPECTIVE...

When I delivered my babies, I was very young (in my 20s and early 30s) and inexperienced. I believed that nothing could possibly go wrong with my pregnancies, so I didn't worry much about what might happen to the baby (or me) if something did go wrong. Fortunately, I was lucky and nothing bad happened.

I have a different perspective with age and experience. Now, I would definitely investigate the neonatal care unit of the hospital, finding out if they had the equipment to treat premature babies or infants with more extreme problems. A level III neonatal unit can treat respiratory problems. A level IV unit can handle any operations (from heart defects to genetic defects) that might occur in your baby.

In the course of five pregnancies, I went to three different hospitals (one private hospital, one teaching hospital, and one woman's hospital) and four different doctors (I finally found the doctor I loved with the fourth child). All of the hospitals turned out to be excellent, but services and care were changing back then, moving toward the L&D rooms that we know today. The best experiences I had were with the last two pregnancies where I had a labor and delivery room, and then a private room after the birth (similar to what you have today). I cherished the privacy and the chance to have real bonding time with my baby and my husband in a hotel-like setting. The pregnancies before that were hospital rooms on a maternity unit.

Another feature that I consider to be important is a lactation nurse to show you how to nurse your baby. Contrary to popular belief, nursing is not something you automatically know how to do. A lot of questions arise while you're attempting to nurse, and problems like cracked nipples and painful breasts can drive you away from nursing and straight to the bottle (baby bottle, that is) if you don't have someone to encourage you and tell you how to handle these issues.

The Absolute Minimum

Don't be "wowed" by extras in a hospital if the actual facilities aren't up to your standards. The bottom line: The hospital might have to save your life or your baby's life. Make sure first and foremost that it is a good hospital with excellent medical facilities. All the rest is gravy....

- Make sure the doctor you want to use can practice at the hospital you choose. Not all doctors have privileges at all hospitals. If the doctor doesn't practice at the hospital of your choice, you're faced with a dilemma—either change doctors or hospitals.
- Visit the hospital ahead of time. Find out where you should go when you're in labor and what you can expect to find when you get there.
- Make sure you know the hospital's rules and procedures. It will make life simpler when you're a patient.
- Pick a hospital that will give you the "birthing" experience that you want, but make sure that it is a quality place with a good medical staff. When all is said and done, it's about safety first.

IN THIS CHAPTER

- How to deal with being pregnant on the job.
- What should you expect from your company with regard to maternity leave?
- Is paternity leave an option?
- Finding and routing out the perfect daycare options.
- Creative ways of going back to work—what are they and how can you make them happen for you?
- Taking care of yourself as a working parent.

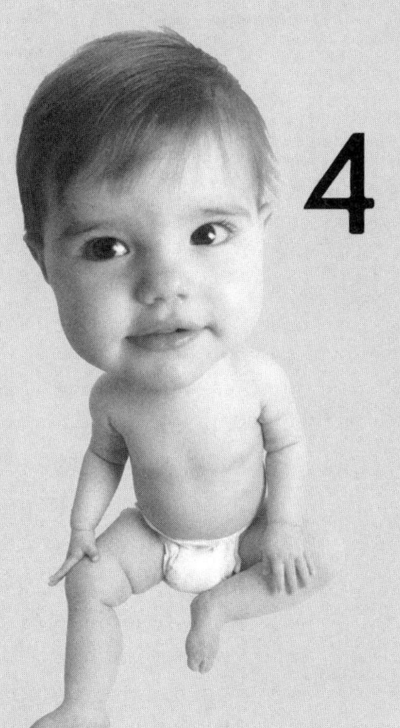

4

DECISIONS THAT AFFECT A WORKING PARENT

If you're a working mother, the advent of a pregnancy presents unique challenges in your life. You'll have to make a lot of decisions that will affect your life and your baby's—and many of those decisions will be gut-wrenching and difficult. Add to that the pressure of working when you're pregnant and tired, and you've got a pressure cooker waiting to explode. Fortunately, many businesses now take the working mother into consideration and help her out with onsite daycare facilities, split schedules/shifts, more flexibility with hours, and shared jobs. Unfortunately, most of those options come *after* the baby is born, so you're usually on your own before the birth.

Dealing with Being Pregnant While Working

The difficulty of being pregnant while holding down a fulltime job is that your life as a working person trudges on, but your body (and mind) may have a hard time keeping up. For example, in the first trimester, you may have to deal with morning sickness. It's not really politic to go rushing out of a meeting or an important phone call to up-chuck. Instead, if you can identify times when you're likely to be sick, then you can try to reschedule meetings or phone calls for a different time of day when you will feel likely better. Also, take preventive measures as much as possible—that is, keep crackers on hand or soda or whatever works to get you through it.

As the pregnancy proceeds, you'll notice that you're more tired, and your feet will start to swell. You can handle these issues by taking short naps during the middle of the day (perhaps the restroom has a couch) or getting outside to take 10-minute walks at break time or whenever possible. Drinking lots of water will increase your profusion of blood to the brain, which will make you feel less tired. . Above all, be kind to yourself and give yourself time off at night when you are at home. Plenty of rest in the evening will go a long way toward making you feel better the next day, and you'll think more clearly.

Put simply—most people will not cut you much slack just because you're pregnant. They will expect you to keep up with your job and pretty much do everything you did before. Your challenge is to figure out how to be kind to yourself but keep up with your responsibilities.

Maternity Leave

Thanks to the Family and Medical Leave Act of 1993 (FMLA), most federal employees are entitled to take a total of up to 12 work weeks of unpaid leave off from their job following the birth of a baby. The good news is that most other major employers have followed suit and apply similar guidelines. (Some large corporations even offer up to a year off—unpaid, of course.) However, be aware that if you are working for a small business of fewer than 50 employees, this act does not apply to you, as it isn't enforced on smaller businesses.

> **tip**
>
> If you apply in writing to your employer requesting FMLA, your company must give you written notice within two business days if you are *not* eligible for FMLA for any reason. If the employer does not respond within two business days, the employee will be eligible to take the leave.

During this time off, you are entitled to receive your benefits, although you may have to pay your share of the costs. Also, your job must be held for you while you are away on leave, or if your job is no longer available when you return, then you must be offered comparable employment.

There are some guidelines, however, that you must follow. You must have worked at least 1,250 hours during a 12-month period prior to taking your leave. And you have to provide a 30-day advance notice for a foreseeable event (which obviously applies to your pregnancy). You also might be asked to provide certification from a medical provider that you are indeed pregnant. You could also be contacted while you are away on maternity leave and asked to verify your status and that you do intend to return to your job.

If you find that you need additional time off due to an emergency with your baby or unexpected circumstances, call your company and ask first before making any assumptions that they can't help you. Often, a company will have an emergency plan in place for just such occurrences.

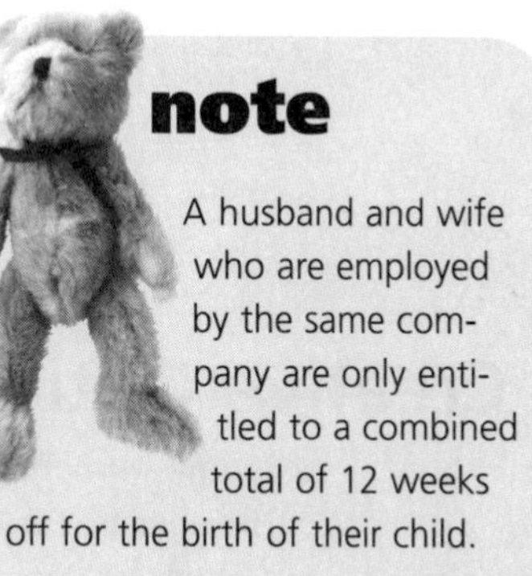

note

A husband and wife who are employed by the same company are only entitled to a combined total of 12 weeks off for the birth of their child.

Receiving Pay While You Are on Maternity Leave

The first thing to do before you get pregnant (preferably) or as soon as you know you are pregnant is to meet with the human resources person in your company to find out what your specific company's policies are for maternity leave and how they apply to you. Each company is different and much will depend on your own circumstances—for example, how long you've been with the company, how much leave you've accrued, and what your position is.

Some companies (usually major corporations) offer full pay and benefits while you are on maternity leave; most do not. In lieu of this, many workers decide to use their sick time or vacation time to be paid while they are on maternity leave, if their employer does not offer compensation during this period. Obviously, if you can build up some cash reserves to use while you're on maternity leave, so much the better.

Paternity Leave

Paternity leave is the time a father takes off after the birth of a child, presumably to help the mother adjust and to bond with his child. Paternity leave is still in its "infancy" stages (pardon the pun). Some companies are quite progressive and offer fathers a paid leave, sometimes as long as six to 12 weeks; however, most companies who offer paternity leave do not necessarily give paid time off. The same stipulations for maternity leave apply to paternity leave in terms of time worked, etc.—the one difference being that if the man is in the highest paid 10 percent bracket of wage earners at his company and the company can show that his absence would cause substantial harm to the organization, then the employer isn't required to keep the job open for the man.

Although more men are beginning to take paternity leave, in some cases, there still might be a stigma attached to it among co-workers or bosses. For this reason, some men are unwilling to take paternity leave, fearing that it could affect their jobs. If your husband is reluctant to take paternity leave, perhaps you can convince him to use some of his vacation time instead.

Creative Options for Going Back to Work

Some women can't wait to go back to work, but most find it difficult to leave their newborns. For this reason, many companies have created job sharing and split schedules. You might want to look into the options available in your particular industry.

If you job share with another person, then you will work part-time, splitting your job with someone else. The benefit is that you get to spend more time at home and are more flexible with your schedule. The downside is that you only make half your normal income, and you might not move up the corporate ladder as quickly. It's also important that you pair up to job share with someone who works in a similar fashion as you do so that you're not stuck doing twice the work in half the time.

Another option might be to telecommute to your job, either all of the time or working from home a specified number of days per week. Many women have opted to do this successfully. If you choose to do this, remember that you are still responsible for actually "being" present in your home office during normal business hours.

Some companies let women work 10-hour days so that they can get more days off in-between—that is, three days off and four days on. If this time is split up over a weekend, there is the potential for your partner to babysit some of those days, thus saving the cost of a sitter.

You also can inquire about flex time (flexible schedules), seeing if you can work odd hours, say a morning schedule from 5 a.m. until 1 in the afternoon or an evening schedule, so that your husband can cover some of the time you would be gone. You never know until you ask what might be possible.

FOR SINGLE MOMS...

No doubt about it—everything is harder for single working mothers. If you're in this situation, try to find some back-up help, whether it is a relative or a family friend. Situations will arise where you simply have to have help. It's best to get it arranged as early as possible *before* the baby comes.

I've been a single working mother, and I don't know how people do it (or how I did it for that matter). But somehow, you just do what needs to be done. If at all possible (and it usually isn't), try to create some space for yourself, particularly some quiet time. Also, negotiate to get away from the baby for a break now and then. No matter how much you love your child, you'll be a better mother for having been away and coming back refreshed. If there is a father in the picture, make sure he has time with the baby. Kids need both parents, assuming that the father is a good parent.

You'll find that you can't always put your kids first ahead of your job, nor can you put the job ahead of your kids. It's a perpetual dilemma because you need to have money to support the kids, but you want to be a good mother. Cut yourself a break and do the best job you can. It's all you can do.

Choosing a Daycare Provider

Choosing a daycare provider when you go back to work can be a nightmare. Take time with this decision and decide in advance what type of facility you want. An ideal situation is to have someone come to your home (i.e., a nanny), but good, qualified people are often difficult to find and can be extremely expensive. If you decide to go this route, make sure you use a reputable agency (if you use one) and do extensive cross-checking of the nanny's references. Most nannies are perfectly safe, but there have been enough cases of child abuse in the news lately to know that there are plenty of deviants out there.

The best alternative might be for a family member or friend to care for your child. But this decision also has positive and negative aspects to it. First, it's difficult to tell someone who is close to you how you want your baby handled. Feelings might get pricked or ruffled, particularly if that person thinks they know all there is to know about babysitting. And it could damage a long-standing friendship if you disagree about how the person handles your child or you are too critical of them. So, be sensitive and informed of the pitfalls before you take this route. And remember that your way is not always the *right* way, but simply *your* way.

Perhaps the most common daycare provider is a certified daycare provider, either in a home or in a stand-alone facility. These facilities should be monitored by the state, which can mean something or nothing, depending on your state and how proactive or overburdened they are.

Here are some questions you might ask a potential sitter for your child:

- What is your philosophy of child rearing?
- Do you punish children? How?
- Do you separate infants from toddler and preschoolers?
- How long have you been in business?
- Could I see a copy of your state license? (It should be displayed in the open.)
- What kind of stimulation do you provide for the children?
- What is your schedule?
- For infants—how often are they held?
- Who are the people you hire to take care of the children? How are they selected?
- What safety precautions do you have or plans for evacuation in case of an emergency or fire.
- May I visit anytime or drop in unexpectedly?
- Do you teach the children, for example, the alphabet or songs?
- Do the children go on field trips?

Base your decision on what you hear and your gut reaction to the place or the people. Never ignore your gut feelings. They are usually right on target.

If you still can't find what you want in a daycare situation, you can always ask around in your workplace or query friends about where they keep their children. If they have older children, ask their kids how they like the place. Kids will always give you an honest answer, sometimes even surprising their own parents.

Your Mental Health and Guilt

Every parent who works feels guilty at one time or another. Here's my best advice: You'll just have to deal with it. Leaving a baby who is crying or ill is one of the hardest things in the world to do. Sometimes, you can take off work and use sick-time to stay home, but more often than not, you have to leave your baby and hope for the best.

The only way to get rid of guilt is to just give it up. It's not worth the time you waste on it.

THE ABSOLUTE MINIMUM

As a working parent, you face obstacles and challenges galore when making your personal life and your job mesh—two areas that are normally at odds with one another. Everyone will seem to want your time, from your boss to your baby to your husband. In the beginning, it's an extremely cumbersome juggling act, but have faith that everything will settle down as you adapt to your new baby, a new way of life, and a new schedule. Impose on your family and friends as much as possible for help and don't be hesitant about taking it. Your baby will be richer for it in the long run.

- Figure out your maternity leave in advance of the birth so that you are not surprised by unexpected glitches in pay or benefits or time off.
- If your husband can get paternity leave, great. If not, ask him to take off as much vacation time or personal time as he feels comfortable with in order to help you adjust to the baby and to give him some bonding time.
- You may be surprised to find that you don't want to return to work in the same way as before, meaning you might prefer part-time work. Investigate your options ahead of time, just in case.
- Shop around for a daycare center or babysitting options as early as possible. Drop in unexpectedly so you get a real sense of how the place is run and how they handle children.
- Take care of yourself mentally and emotionally by scheduling some time off. You are the baby's most important caretaker. Make sure you don't burn out with the pressure of working fulltime and being a new mother.

PART II

Now That You're Pregnant First Trimester

IN THIS CHAPTER

- Identifying physical changes
- Causes of some of the problems
- Relieving the symptoms when possible
- Dealing with emotional issues

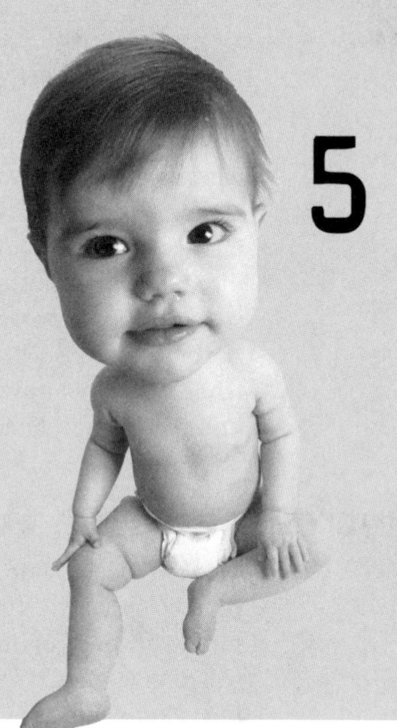

5

FIRST TRIMESTER—MOTHER

From a physiological standpoint, many body changes occur in the first three months, most of them invisible to the naked eye. But even if other people can't tell that you're pregnant, you'll know for sure. You'll feel "different" as your body starts its journey "prepping" for and "cocooning" that growing baby inside you.

First, there will be a surge in hormones associated with the pregnancy, affecting many organ systems including the uterus. Next, the uterus starts to change by growing and adapting to the pregnancy, although you will not perceive any growth in the stomach area for several months. If everything is normal, the cells will continue to grow and divide while the baby forms. Here are some other systemic and psychological changes you might experience.

note

Note that the uterus is rotated slightly to the right due to some anatomical changes. This leads to more compression of the right ureter, which in turn increases the dilation of the right ureter. If you were to get an infection of the kidney (although both kidneys and both sides can be affected), it's more likely to hurt on the right side, and you'll notice pain on the right side of your back if that happens. Also, it's fairly common for pregnant women to have urinary tract infections (commonly known as *UTIs*), characterized by that burning sensation when you urinate. Most of these infections are caught early while it is localized to the bladder and treated with a simple course of oral antibiotics. If allowed to progress, however, the infection can rise via the ureters themselves. Kidney infections can be dangerous for both mother and baby. Get treatment immediately if you suspect an infection.

Increased Urine Output

This is a biggie, since it's something you'll notice right away. As the pregnancy progresses, the mother's blood volume will expand. The kidneys will receive more blood flow and at a faster rate as the volume increases by about 50%. The increases in both blood volume and flow rate result in a better profusion of all the organ systems, especially the uterus. As the kidneys experience the increased blood volume at a faster rate, urine production is increased also.

Translation for mothers: You're going to have to go to the bathroom a lot. This blood flow and subsequent urine production is a gradual process that increases throughout the pregnancy.

Congestion

Another change that you might notice is feeling as if you have a cold or are congested. This condition results from the mucus membranes becoming swollen and mucous production being more pronounced as the hormonal changes associated with pregnancy occur.

Some women may think they have a cold and go to the doctor to get it checked out. There is really not a whole lot you can do except to live with this condition. Taking nasal decongestants or antihistamines is not advisable since you don't really have a cold, and you don't want to take the unnecessary risk of hurting the fetus. Occasionally, symptoms may warrant the use of medications, but check with your doctor first. It varies how long this congestion lasts—it could last anywhere from a few weeks to the entire pregnancy. This isn't usually a serious or debilitating problem that most women complain about—it's just something to be noticed.

caution

This warning is obvious—don't ever get too far away from any bathroom facilities. When the urge strikes, ya gotta go. Control is out the window when you're pregnant.

Morning Sickness

Morning sickness is probably the best-known symptom of early pregnancy—and there are few things worse than that telltale queasiness and the subsequent rushing to the *john* (apologies to Dr. John for the use of his name in vain). No one is exactly sure what triggers morning sickness, but it is thought that it occurs due to hormonal elevation. Fortunately for humanity, most symptoms subside by the end of the first trimester.

tip

Surprisingly, congestion can also be an early symptom of pregnancy. It's not uncommon for women to think they have a cold but to have morning sickness and be pregnant instead.

Morning sickness, despite its reference to "morning," can occur any time of the day, and some people experience it all day long. Oddly enough, there is no data suggesting that more women experience morning sickness in the morning. Personally, I don't ever remember experiencing morning sickness in the morning—it was always in the afternoon.

Anything can bring on morning sickness from a simple smell or odor from a food (or odors from perfume, trash, ...you name it). Chances are that you might feel queasiness coming on after you taste a certain food or beverage. In my case, caffeine always did it for me—just the smell or taste of coffee or coke or any caffeine substance, and I felt the bile rising and the urge to up-chuck.

The general rule of thumb in combating morning sickness is to *listen,* really listen, to your body. If you feel you can't eat a particular food, then focus primarily on hydration, in other words, push fluids into your body. And don't eat until you feel better (with the obvious qualification that you *have* to eat something sometime). But don't just drink any liquids—focus on consuming more clear liquids rather than milk, for example. Some people can tolerate milk, but often it just worsens your nausea. You should know fairly quickly whether or not milk works for you. (Keep in mind that after the morning sickness goes away, which it should as the pregnancy progresses, you can add milk or other foods back into your diet.)

DEFINING A CLEAR LIQUID

If you can hold a glass up and read a newspaper behind it, it's a clear liquid. Generally, we're referring to water, Gatorade, Sprite, ginger-ale, Mello Yello, clear soups, and so forth.

Also stay away from rich foods and sauces, which tend to exacerbate morning sickness. If you have a craving or develop a preference for a specific food, go ahead and eat it. To combat symptoms of morning sickness, women can try eating crackers, breads, or gingersnaps—anything that sounds good and that you can tolerate (meaning it doesn't come back up).

In terms of prenatal vitamins, all pregnant women should be taking vitamins, especially if they're sick a lot. However, prenatal vitamins actually can cause women to be sick or contribute to their nausea. In that situation, try a different prenatal vitamin made by a different manufacturer or perhaps take a Flintstones vitamin (all humor aside—it's better than nothing). Once the symptoms improve, go back on your prenatal vitamin.

THAT CAFFEINE "FIX"

It's probably okay to drink caffeine, but it's not something that doctors encourage women to drink in large quantities. Try to limit your caffeine intake to one cup of coffee or tea a day or one can of soda. Although caffeine consumption hasn't been shown to have long-term adverse effects on the baby (at least not in studies thus far), it can act as a diuretic for the mother, and losing water isn't good for the mother or the baby.

It's not clear whether a diet high in proteins or complex carbohydrates helps with morning sickness. Eat as normally as possible, and "liberate" your food and liquid choices (a Dr. John term, meaning add them back into your diet—can food really be liberated?) as you can tolerate things.

Vomiting

If you're throwing up constantly, the doctor will rule out obvious causes first; for example if there is an inciting food or drug/medicine you're taking that's causing the vomiting. Keep in mind that vomiting isn't always caused by pregnancy. You might simply have the flu or other viral infection, or some kind of gastro-intestinal disorder unrelated to pregnancy. In rare cases, vomiting may be caused by an abnormal pregnancy or other abnormal hormonal condition and should be checked out by the doctor.

caution

Don't try any over-the-counter substances of any kind without first consulting with your doctor!

The doctor may prescribe an anti-emetic (anti-nausea) medicine for you; however, in general, most doctors will try nonprescription methods first because it's less risky to the developing pregnancy. There are certain over-the-counter remedies that work occasionally, including ginger supplements. Sometimes, a doctor may recommend a vitamin B-6 tablet combined with Unisom, which is a brand-name sleeping aid. It's considered fairly safe unless there is a medical contraindication to taking it.

If none of the above options work, the doctor may prescribe a prescription strength medication, such as Phenergan or Compazine, Reglan, or Zofran. Any one of these four drugs usually helps most women get through their nauseous period.

In rare cases or if all else fails, a woman might be admitted to the hospital for IV fluids and medications given through an IV (particularly if she can't keep medicine down). Other possible causes for extreme vomiting could include being pregnant with twins, having a thyroid abnormality, or having a molar pregnancy (where the pregnancy grows abnormally). The latter cases will usually be treated with medication or surgery.

Shortness of Breath

Some women complain about shortness of breath during the first trimester (or beyond). This condition could be caused either by hormonal changes or by the diaphragm being elevated due to the growing pregnancy so that it restricts the downward movement that allows a woman to expand her lungs. Sometimes, women may have a perception that they are having trouble breathing, but in fact, they are fine, and there is usually nothing about which to be concerned. If a shortness of breath occurs, the remedy is to stay calm and not panic. Take a few deep breaths and relax. Generally, that anxious feeling will pass, and your breathing will resume normally.

However, if you have a prepregnancy pulmonary condition like asthma before becoming pregnant or develop it while you're pregnant (which does happen), this condition could possibly be exacerbated with pregnancy, and you should consult your doctor immediately. Asthma is not something to fool around with at any time.

Get help quickly if you are an asthmatic. Check with your doctor to see which medicines you can use while pregnant.

Anemia

There is a physiologic anemia that begins early in pregnancy and is considered normal. While it's not really a true anemia in the classic sense—but rather a *physiologic* anemia, meaning that it only occurs in pregnancy—it still needs to be treated. What happens is that there is a 50% increase in an expectant mother's plasma volume, but only about a 20–40% increase in her red blood cells. This discrepancy leads to a dilutional effect. The body *thinks* it is anemic because of this dilutional effect, and the result is that the woman does actually feel tired. Because of this relative anemia, most physicians in the U.S. give pregnant women prenatal vitamin supplements that contain the necessary iron that she might lack. However, rarely will a woman require more iron than can be found in the normal prenatal vitamin. Her anemic status will be checked again in the third trimester, and additional iron supplements may be added at that time as needed.

note

In ancient times it was thought that women were sick in the first trimester because it kept them from eating or drinking potentially dangerous foods in the early stages of pregnancy. It's probably an old wive's tale, but it does make for some interesting conversations among doctors. Doctors still speculate whether or not this could be true from an evolutionary standpoint. Personally, I think the doctors could be a bit more creative about this. I think morning sickness evolved so that women wouldn't be tempted to have a baby every year. If it were totally delightful, we'd be overpopulated. And that's probably why labor is so darn hard, too.

Other "Icky" Body Changes

Some other common symptoms or complaints during the first trimester are as follows:

- Heartburn and indigestion
- Weight gain
- Constipation
- Backaches
- Headaches
- Faintness or dizziness

caution

Always avoid environmental exposure to smoke, whether caused by cigarettes or fires. Not only could the smoke affect your breathing, but the toxins are also dangerous for your baby.

- Fatigue and stress
- Increased vaginal discharge
- Breast discomfort due to enlargement
- Complexion problems
- Venous changes

Heartburn and Indigestion

In the case of heartburn or indigestion, conservative efforts are key. Before rushing to the doctor for medication, try to sort through the condition on your own. First, think about what you're eating and avoid foods that give you heartburn, such as foods or drinks that have carbonation or rich sauces or juices that would increase gastric acid production. Also, don't eat too close to bedtime or naptime. The recumbent position stimulates acid reflux and increases heartburn. Try a fairly bland diet for a while and drink lots of water.

note

Over the counter antacids are probably safe in the short run, but since no thorough medical studies have been done on these drugs, it's probably better to check with your doctor first.

Weight Gain

Some weight gain, particularly around the waist, is normal. However, if you're gaining an inordinate amount of weight in the first trimester, consult with your doctor. First, make sure you are not pregnant with multiple gestations (i.e., twins). Next, try to rule out any physiological reason for the weight gain, such as any pre-existing medical condition or hormonal disorder (possibly thyroid disease, diabetes, or Cushing's disease or syndrome). Make sure you're eating a healthful diet with the requisite amounts of fruits, vegetables, proteins, and complex carbohydrates. Try to cut out excess sugar and calories, such as fried foods and fast foods. The first trimester is not the time to gain weight. An ideal weight gain for this period would likely be based on your body mass index (BMI), which can be calculated using your prepregnancy height and weight (see Figure 5.1). These calculations can be performed at your doctor's office, and at that time an estimate for an appropriate weight gain can be determined. However, for the average American woman, the ideal weight gain in the first half of pregnancy would be 5–7 pounds.

FIGURE 5.1

Here are two examples of BMI charts that health care providers use as a reference point. Of course, these charts are not for pregnant women, so you'll have to figure out where you started prepregnancy and go from there.

$$\text{BMI}=\left\{\frac{\text{WEIGHT(pounds)}}{\text{HEIGHT(inches)}}\right\}\times 703$$

Weight in Pounds

Height in Feet and Inches	120	130	140	150	160	170	180	190	200	210	220	230	240	250
4'6	29	31	34	36	39	41	43	46	48	51	53	56	58	60
4'8	27	29	31	34	36	38	40	43	45	47	49	52	54	56
4'10	25	27	29	31	34	36	38	40	42	44	46	48	50	52
5'0	23	25	27	29	31	33	35	37	39	41	43	45	47	49
5'2	22	24	26	27	29	31	33	35	37	38	40	42	44	46
5'4	21	22	24	26	28	29	31	33	34	36	38	40	41	43
5'6"	19	21	23	24	26	27	29	31	32	34	36	37	39	40
5'8	18	20	21	23	24	26	27	29	30	32	34	35	37	38
5'10	17	19	20	22	23	24	26	27	29	30	32	33	35	36
6'0	16	18	19	20	22	23	24	26	27	28	30	31	33	34
6'2"	15	17	18	19	21	22	23	24	26	27	28	30	31	32
6'4	15	16	17	18	20	21	22	23	24	26	27	28	29	30
6'6	14	15	16	17	19	20	21	22	23	24	25	27	28	29
6'8	13	14	15	17	18	19	20	21	22	23	24	25	26	28

Healthy Weight | Overweight | Obese

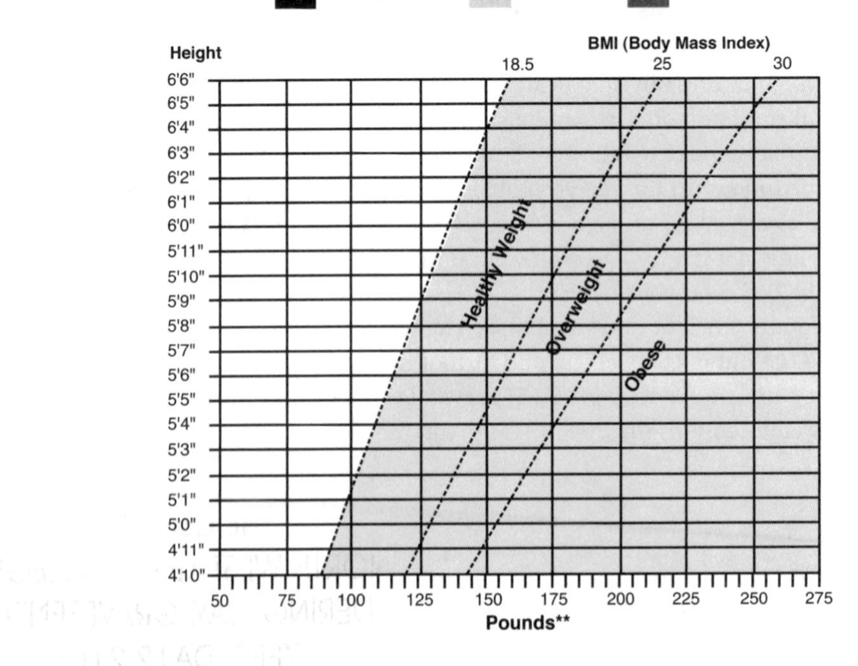

Constipation

Constipation occurs because the intestines have less motility due to hormonal changes. What this means is that the intestines are not pushing the fecal matter through the bowel as efficiently as before the pregnancy. Therefore, the stools become drier as the water in them is reabsorbed by the intestines, which leads to firmer and drier stools, and the unpleasant feeling associated with constipation.

The remedy is to drink lots of fluids (preferably water) and watch what you eat. Don't eat a lot of cheese and greasy foods. If you can increase your fiber intake, so much the better. Try eating a good bran cereal in the morning and drink juice at that time as well. If these remedies don't work, your doctor may need to prescribe a stool softener.

Backaches

Backaches are pretty common in pregnancy. They are caused by the stress and strain on the muscles that support the lower back and pelvic region. There are also mechanical issues involved. As your center of gravity moves forward, you'll lean backwards to compensate from flailing forward. Naturally, this creates an increased amount of strain on the back muscles. In addition, there are hormonal changes, specifically a hormone called *relaxin*, which is produced by the body and helps to loosen the ligaments and attachments in the pelvic region in order to accommodate the baby. All of these things, plus poor posture and possibly poor physical conditioning, can increase a person's risk for back pain. The basic physiological change that is occurring is an inflammatory response to the strain-induced muscle and back injury.

> **caution**
>
> Normally when you're not pregnant, a doctor would recommend rest and an anti-inflammatory drug, such as Motrin or Aleve, but in pregnancy this is not advised, as these medicines have been known to be potentially harmful. These types of medicines can have a toxic effect on a fetus's developing kidneys, which can affect the amount of amniotic fluid that is produced. And later in pregnancy, these meds can affect the baby's heart and the circulation of blood.

To relieve back pain, try some gentle stretching exercises in the morning and evening. Work on having good posture during the day and use a support pillow propped behind your lower back in an ergonomic chair if you are working at a desk. Take more frequent breaks to walk around and stretch—at least once an hour. If you have to lift something, make sure that you lift properly so you don't aggravate the back problem. Don't bend over; rather, squat down and lift with your legs and not your back.

Your partner or significant other can be a big help here. Have him apply a warm compress or heating pad (or warm towel) to the back and massage it through the towel. You can also take a warm bath—anything that soothes the area.

In addition, sometimes taking Tylenol or acetaminophen may help, as long as you don't have a medical reason not to take these medicines. For some people, it may be appropriate to use a back brace or pregnancy girdle. Check with your doctor and make sure these devices do not constrict the abdomen too tightly.

tip

Stomach muscles support the back. If you have good, strong stomach muscles before the pregnancy (i.e., you've done lots of crunches, etc.), you will probably have fewer back problems during pregnancy. Once you're pregnant, however, exercise caution when attempting any stomach exercises.

Headaches

Headaches can be pretty common in the first trimester, and often migraines are a problem for women who have had a pre-existing diagnosis (Figure 5.2). Again, conservative treatment is key. Identify the behavior that creates the headache if you can; for example, not enough sleep or not enough hydration, the wrong kinds of food, stress, or whatever. Try to alleviate the problem first. If that doesn't work, you can consider taking Tylenol or using cold compresses on your forehead. If nothing seems to help, see your physician.

note

Bright lights (or sunlight) can trigger headaches easily in women who are prone to migraines. Turn the lights down while inside; wear sunglasses while outside.

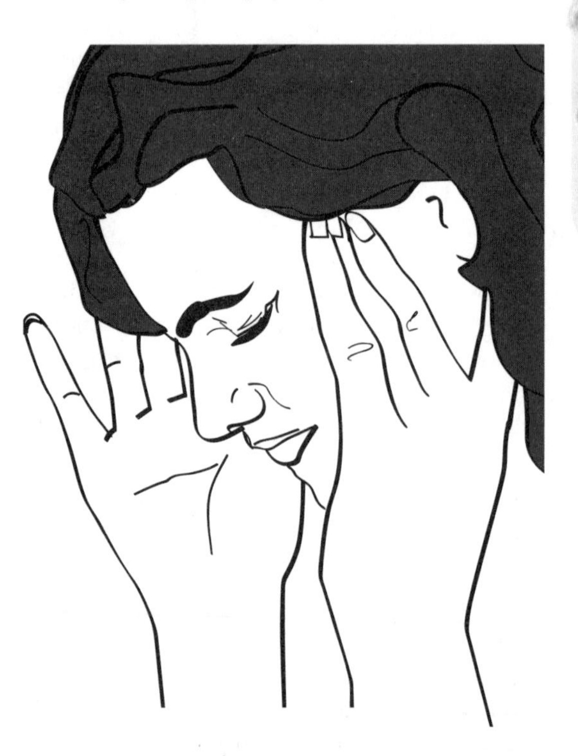

FIGURE 5.2
In some women, pregnancy can make a headache or migraine even worse.

Faintness or Dizziness

During pregnancy, women can be more prone to a vagal reaction, which is a neurological reaction that dilates blood vessels leading to the brain and lowers the blood pressure temporarily causing a feeling of light-headedness. To combat feeling faint or dizzy, be careful about standing up too suddenly or making sudden changes in positions (from lying down to getting up too quickly). Again, make sure that you're drinking plenty of fluids to offset this condition. Women who aren't properly hydrated are more sensitive to this blood pressure drop.

Fatigue and Stress

Being tired is a common complaint that most pregnant women have, and it's understandable. Because being pregnant is full of changes to your health, you should expect moments of fatigue and plan for them. Don't expect your life to go on as it did before with the same degree of energy. Anticipate this exhausted condition because it *will* happen. By anticipating, you can better prepare yourself for the change and make some effort to make lifestyle changes to compensate for fatigue, such as adjusting your sleep and work schedule accordingly.

HIBERNATION

Fatigue is the one thing I remember most about my first trimester, particularly in my first pregnancy. I felt like a bear because all I wanted to do was hibernate and sleep. My husband went to work, and I crawled back to bed and slept. I slept until lunch. I slept some more in the afternoon. Then I slept all night. It was the strangest feeling—always being tired. Fortunately, it mysteriously disappeared one day, and I regained most of my energy

Stress isn't good for you or the baby. Stress can cause all kinds of symptoms from headaches to anxiety to depression to affecting your immune system in a negative way. Stress also makes you more prone to infections (for example, colds, UTIs, and so on).

There are two kinds of stress. One kind is productive—it's the kind that motivates you to achieve goals or objectives, keeps you on time, and allows you to accomplish your tasks. This type of stress can be a good thing. But the other kind of stress is the kind that is defeating and keeps you from focusing and from achieving everything you need to do—it's the opposite of the first type. This stress is counterproductive to your ability to manage affairs in your life or to maintain your health. These are the kinds of stressors that should be looked at more closely, and you should strive to reduce them and the situation that is causing the stress.

Increased Vaginal Discharge

An increased vaginal discharge is not unusual for pregnant women because it is caused by hormonal changes involving the cervix and vagina. In fact, women should expect to have more discharge coming from the vagina. In most cases, this is nothing that will pose a problem or interfere with your lifestyle, but vaginal discharge should *not* be confused with an infection. If you think you are having signs of an infection, for example, foul odor, pain, irritation, or bleeding, this could represent an infection, and you should see your doctor for an evaluation.

Breast Discomfort Due to Enlargement

Breast discomfort is pretty common among pregnant women as the breast stretches and enlarges in order to accommodate future lactation. In fact, some women will suspect they are pregnant because their breasts hurt. Other women experience more discomfort closer to delivery. For many women, the pain varies from the beginning of the pregnancy until the end. It can feel like a brief, shooting pain or a dull ache.

The most important thing you can do to alleviate the pain is to wear a good support bra and pay attention to any skin changes, like cracked nipples or irritated skin, which may require some form of treatment. Treatment is usually not necessary, but ointments can be prescribed that may help alleviate the symptoms.

note

Enlarged breasts can also contribute to back pain, so the good supportive bra becomes even more important. This is not the place to skimp when it comes to money. Buy the best maternity bra that you can find, regardless of the cost.

While most breast pain is fairly common and normal, it can also be an indicator of something being wrong with your breast (possibly an early tumor). Always tell your doctor if you are worried or the pain is out of the ordinary or unbearable.

Complexion Problems

Ever hear that a woman who is pregnant glows? In some cases, a woman's complexion and skin actually look better during pregnancy, almost as if she is glowing. However, other women may develop a condition called *chloasma* (a darkening of the skin), which is also known as the "mask of pregnancy." Basically, it's a facial pigmentation caused by an increase in estrogen and progesterone. Also, those same hormonal changes can cause hyper pigmentation in other areas, for example, a line around the belly-button and darkening of the nipple area (areola) and perineum. Not to worry—usually these changes will fade after the delivery.

Venous (Vein) Changes

As pregnancy progresses, there is a decrease in vascular resistance, potentially relaxing the veins, which then can lead to a greater likelihood for hemorrhoids or varicose veins. There isn't too much you can do about this, and it doesn't affect everyone. If you're having trouble with constipation, this can cause hemorrhoids. You can wear support hose for varicose veins, as long as they don't go over the stomach. Consult your doctor if either condition becomes unbearable.

Emotional Changes

The emotional changes that occur in the first trimester can run the gamut from extreme happiness to extreme sadness, some of it depending on how you view your pregnancy. Don't be surprised by this roller coaster of emotions—it's natural with the hormonal changes that are occurring. Try to get plenty of sleep, since being tired can cause additional stress and more emotional upheaval.

Surprisingly, some women have more energy during this time period, simply because they are happier. For the most part, however, women are less energetic because their body changes make them feel more tired.

Remember that pregnancy does not solve any family problems you might have, and sometimes it can add to them. If you need to talk to someone, there are plenty of people available to help. You can look for support groups on the Internet or ask your doctor for references—and don't forget your clergy if you're so inclined. The important thing is to get help and not to try to tough it out alone.

caution

Again, if you have any symptoms of depression, consult your physician immediately. Anti-depressant medication may be taken during the pregnancy, but this needs to be discussed with your doctor.

Along with all the other things going on, physical changes can cause women to feel unhappy with their body image, perhaps making them feel less attractive. Contrary to what most women believe, Dr. John assures me that many men think that there are few things more beautiful than a woman who is pregnant. Just remember that beauty does come from within, and if you're happy, generally the world around you is happy. Remind yourself that you are pregnant, not fat, and your body will change back to normal after the delivery. Plus, you'll have a baby as an added bonus! The result is worth the temporary shift in your body image.

THE ABSOLUTE MINIMUM

The first trimester brings with it a whole host of changes to the pregnant woman—all coming at once. It can be disconcerting at best; overwhelming at worst. Our philosophy is that if you're prepared for what is coming, it will be easier to face and adjust to the extreme changes.

- Depending on your pregnancy, the physical changes could be great or subtle, but you *will* notice a difference in your body.
- Many of the body changes in the first trimester are easy to live with and shouldn't upset your routine much.
- If you are one of the women who have a miserable time physically the first trimester, then talk to your health care professional and get help. Help is only a phone call away. Don't tough it out—it's not necessary.
- Always, always trust your gut intuition. If you think something is wrong, call your doctor or midwife.
- It would be downright surprising if you didn't have any emotional ups and downs during this period. The pregnancy aside—simply adjusting to the fact that you're going to have a baby can cause a lot of stress. Talk to people about your feelings and get a support group in place. If that doesn't help, enlist the care of a professional.

In This Chapter

- What does the baby look like at this early stage?
- What is formed in the baby; what isn't?
- What can be harmful to the fetus in the first trimester?

6

First Trimester—Baby

As you're changing and growing, so is the baby inside of you. It's difficult to imagine just how much growth is packed into such a short period of time. In the first three months, the fetus is only 8–10 millimeters in length (the width of your thumb), but within that embryo is a beating heart with blood circulating through it and the potential for growth with the maturation of multiple organ systems. At this point, it's difficult to determine the gender, but limb buds that will eventually change and become arms and legs are clearly visible. Doctors can also identify the cranial (head) portion of the fetus. They will use this crown-rump length from an ultrasound (roughly the distance between the head portion of the embryo and its bottom side) as a form of measurement to determine how far along the pregnancy is. It's actually fairly accurate when measured.

Physiological Changes in the Baby's Growth

When the sperm meets the egg, a virtual explosion occurs in terms of rapid cellular division. By the end of the first trimester, most of the baby's organ systems are formed, including the heart, lungs, kidneys, and digestive system. Still forming is the baby's neurological system, including the brain, brain stem, and spinal cord. Organ formation occurs through most of the first trimester. Afterwards, the organ systems that have formed are increasing in size and maturation

> **note**
>
> The medical term for the increase in the number of cells is *hyperplasia*. It occurs primarily in the first trimester.
>
> *Hypertrophy* is the growth of the cells that have already formed. This change generally occurs after the first trimester and lasts throughout the pregnancy.

By about the fifth or sixth week of pregnancy, heart motion is visible with a trans-vaginal ultrasound, although most of the other systems are too small to see at this time. A fluid sac has developed around the fetus that will eventually comprise the amniotic fluid. The yolk sac is present in early pregnancy, although it slowly regresses and the placenta takes its place as the major support system of nutrients and the exchange of waste products.

INCIDENCE OF MISCARRIAGE

The incidence of miscarriage in the first three months is high—from 30–40%; however, this figure might actually be higher because many cases are unidentified or underreported. For example, some women may actually be pregnant and not realize it when they have abnormal bleeding. Because some of these pregnancies are mistaken for abnormal menstrual bleeding, the diagnosis of pregnancy is missed and thus underreported. This is not to imply that all abnormal periods are due to a pregnancy, but it might explain some of the reported discrepancies.

Products That Can Affect the Fetus

The mother's body acts as a holding vehicle for the fetus while it develops. Because the mother and baby are so intricately intertwined, good and bad substances can traverse the placenta. In other words, what affects the mother, usually affects the baby.

Sometimes, we inadvertently expose ourselves to something harmful. Accidents do happen; however, there are many substances that we *know* in advance are harmful, and yet we still continue to use them. The two most obvious products to avoid are tobacco and alcohol, but there are others that can be equally damaging. Make sure that you know the risks and think twice before you expose your baby to some of these dangerous substances.

Tobacco

The use of tobacco during pregnancy has been extensively studied. It's been proven that smoking tobacco products during pregnancy can have a bad effect on the fetus. Even limited or minimal exposure to cigarette smoke (second-hand) can have adverse effects on the fetus.

The effects on the fetus include:

- A noticeable increase in babies with low birth weight (intra-uterine growth restriction)
- An increased risk for fetal anomalies (abnormal development)
- An increased risk of still-births

WHY IS LOW BIRTH WEIGHT HARMFUL?

Low birth rate is a serious problem because it can impact the baby's future growth and development. Babies who are unusually small in size and weight pose the greatest risks for developmental and cognitive disabilities, visual problems that can lead to blindness, and chronic lung disease.

Low birth weight can be caused by pre-term labor, but cigarette smoking, as well as poor nutrition, have also been linked with an increasing prevalence of low birth weight babies.

However, babies can also be small for constitutional reasons, for example, it's their genetic predisposition for size and weight. This type of low birth weight does not usually pose a problem for the baby's growth and development.

Besides affecting the baby in a harmful way, smoking tobacco also affects the mother's health during pregnancy in many ways:

- Smoking has been linked with pulmonary or lung problems. As we mentioned previously, breathing during pregnancy can already be compromised and tobacco can worsen that condition. Mucous production can be increased as a result of inflammation of the bronchial tree, which can lead to increased coughing and irritation of the pulmonary lining.
- If you have a pre-existing pulmonary condition, such as asthma, using tobacco can worsen this situation and make standard treatment less effective.
- Tobacco can adversely impact your immune system so you are more likely to develop infections, such as pneumonia or viral illnesses.
- As the immune system is compromised, there is an increased risk for cervical abnormalities, including precancerous changes known as *dysplasia*, which can affect the outcome of the pregnancy.
- A woman may have nutritional deficiencies associated with smoking because she's not eating as well.
- Tobacco not only impacts a woman during her pregnancy but can also affect her postpartum recovery period; for example, healing from a C-section or episiotomy repair is less effective because the body's healing abilities are compromised.
- Smoking can adversely affect the quality of blood flow that reaches the uterus and the fetus. Any reduction in blood volume can directly affect the potential growth of the fetus.
- Toxins in the blood as a result of cigarette smoking can reduce the amount of oxygen that is available to the baby.

The good news is that the message is finally getting out to pregnant women that smoking is bad for them, and the incidence of pregnant women who smoke appears to be declining (see Figure 6.1).

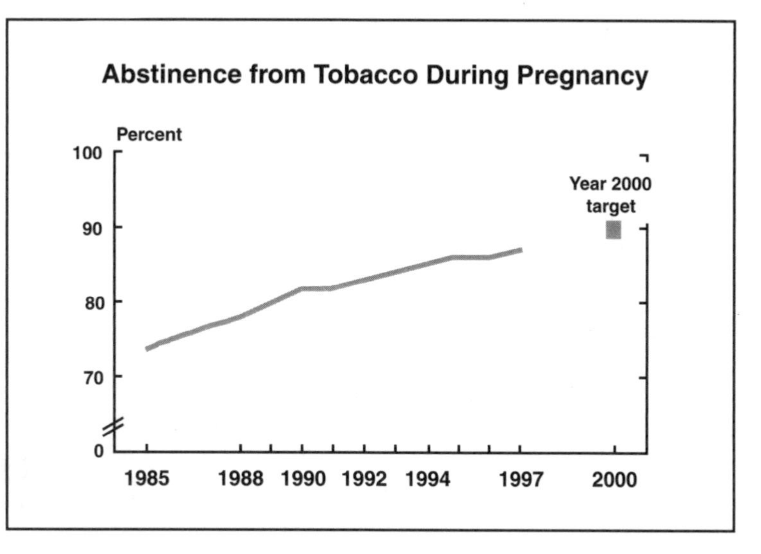

FIGURE 6.1
Fortunately, as the chart shows, more women are refraining from smoking every year.

Alcohol

Alcohol is the most commonly abused drug of choice for women. Drinking alcohol during the first trimester can undermine the baby's health by undermining the mother's health. A pregnant woman who drinks can't take in as much folic acid or thiamine in her body as necessary, which can lead to malnutrition for both mother and baby. Drinking alcohol during pregnancy also increases the mother's chances for liver disease, pneumonia, bone marrow suppression, and miscarriages. A more obvious risk is the risk for trauma associated with accidents caused by being intoxicated.

caution

Driving and drinking is dangerous at any time, but when you are pregnant, the risk to your baby increases one hundred-fold. If you are in an accident while pregnant, you run the risk of injuring the fetus.

Even more importantly, drinking alcohol can damage the baby's health permanently. Because alcohol crosses the placenta, a baby's blood level for alcohol can mimic or approximate the mother's blood alcohol level. Babies born to alcoholic mothers frequently have fetal alcohol syndrome, which is a manifestation of alcohol exposure in utero. The incidence of fetal alcohol syndrome appears to be on the rise (see Figure 6.2).

Babies born with fetal alcohol syndrome have a greater incidence of mental retardation. They frequently have central nervous system problems, as well as facial features that may look different than other babies. Often, they have developmental problems with their organ systems, including the kidneys and the heart. In some cases, fetal alcohol syndrome even causes death.

The amount of alcohol considered to be safe in pregnancy is unknown. For that reason, physicians recommend abstinence.

caution

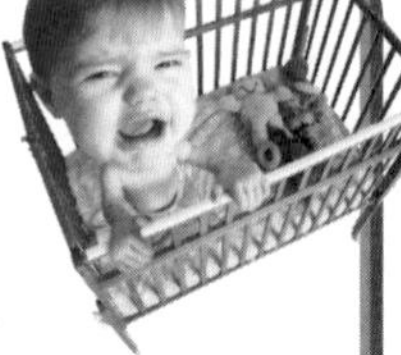

The risk of miscarriage is increased two to four-fold in women who drink.

If someone were to have four drinks a day, approximately 30% of the babies born would have fetal alcohol syndrome. Another 30% would show some prenatal toxic effect.

Medicine

Not surprisingly, there are very few studies available in medical literature that test the effects of medicine on the fetus. For obvious ethical and moral reasons, testing has not been sanctioned on human pregnancies. Therefore, physicians are somewhat limited in their knowledge regarding specific effects of medications on unborn babies. The information they do have is based mostly on anecdotal evidence (opinions based on what they've observed) or on controlled studies performed on animals. Granted, testing animals is not the greatest way to test the effects of drugs on humans, but it's the only method we've got at the moment. Unfortunately, it can be fraught with potential errors.

note

The reality is that often women who smoke or drink regularly in their everyday lives may find out they are pregnant after they've had contact with these products. The best advice is to stop using tobacco and alcohol if you plan on getting pregnant, or the minute you find out you are pregnant. Although it's unclear what damage may have been caused already, you can minimize your future risk. The sooner you stop, the better.

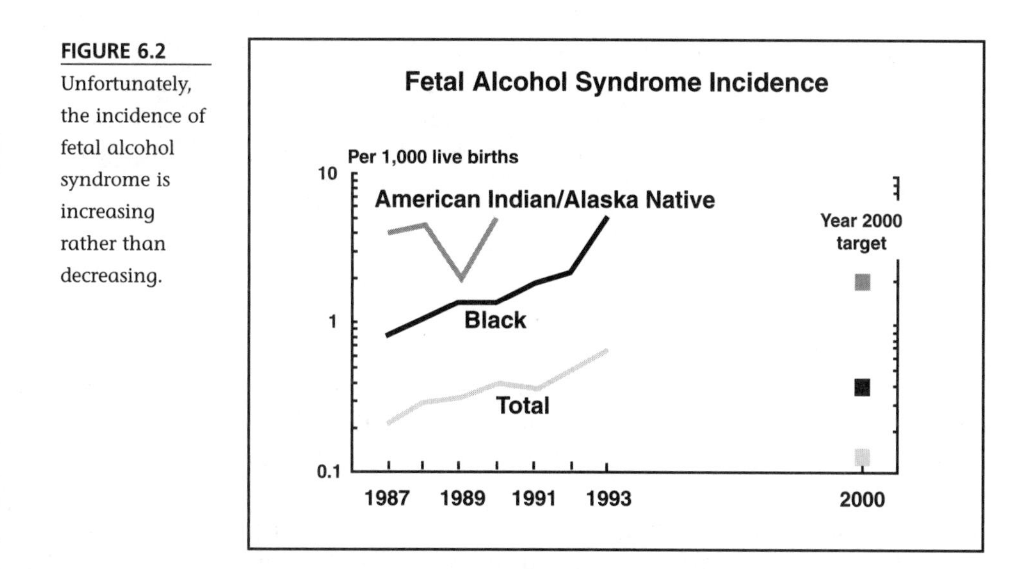

FIGURE 6.2 Unfortunately, the incidence of fetal alcohol syndrome is increasing rather than decreasing.

HOW THE DOCTORS MEASURE THE EFFECTS OF DRUGS

Physicians use the *Physicians Desk Reference* as a guide for the effects of drugs on the human body. The FDA has established five categories for drugs and medications with regards to possible adverse effects on the fetus. These five categories include: A,B,C,D, and X.

An A rating means that controlled studies in humans have demonstrated no fetal risks (examples would include prenatal vitamins). Most medicines taken by pregnant women fall into the B and C range. Category B indicates that animals showed no fetal risks when tested, but that there weren't any controlled studies of the drug done on humans (an example of a B drug would be penicillin). Category C indicates that risks to humans have not been ruled out, but that there are no adequate studies that have been done (examples might include over-the-counter cold medicines). With a rating of D, there is evidence of fetal risk, but the benefits are thought to outweigh the risks (examples would be certain anti-seizure medicines). A rating of "X" means that you absolutely don't want to give this medication to a pregnant woman (an example would be Retin A).

Always be careful and consult with your doctor first before taking any over-the-counter or prescription medications. Doctors can determine if the risk benefit ratio makes it worth taking.

So, for what it's worth, here is what the doctors have deduced. Don't take any unnecessary medications during the first trimester. Avoid all aspirin products, Motrin products, and antibiotics, unless you have a good reason for taking them. If a woman is *on* anti-depressants and can get *off* them, then that is probably better for the baby. However, if the risk of *not* taking an anti-depressant for the mother is greater than the risk to the baby, then she should probably continue taking them. (For example, if the mother has a history of suicidal thoughts and the meds are helping, then she should keep taking them.)

Illegal Drugs

Simply put—they're bad. In general, the same concerns that you have for cigarette smoking apply to all illegal drugs.

One of the major problems with babies born to mothers who have taken addictive medications or drugs (such as cocaine or heroin) is that the baby can undergo withdrawal problems just like the mother. When it manifests in the baby, it's called *neonatal abstinence syndrome*. Classic symptoms of this disorder in the baby include central nervous system irritability, gastro-intestinal dysfunction, respiratory disorders or distress, shakes or tremors, high-pitched crying, poor feeding, and electrolyte disturbances. Anyone who has seen a "crack baby" knows the signs—the baby acts as if it is in constant distress and can't be comforted. It's a horrible condition to inflict on a baby.

Statistics show that approximately 10–15% of the women of childbearing age in urban centers are using cocaine during pregnancy. When cocaine is introduced into the pregnant woman's body, it prevents the removal or uptake of norepinephrine (adrenaline). This causes an increase in vascular constriction in the mother, which translates to a faster heartbeat and a rapid rise in both the maternal and fetal blood pressures. Consequently, uterine and placental blood flow decrease because of the vascular constriction, which then results in a rapid fetal heart rate and increased fetal oxygen consumption. Uterine contractions can also increase. The danger is that there is a significant risk factor for placental abruption, which is a premature separation of placenta from the uterus, and can lead to the baby's death if not treated immediately in the hospital.

caution

Cocaine used in the first trimester can increase the risk of spontaneous abortion or miscarriage by about 40 50%. There is also a 15 20% incidence of SIDS (sudden infant death syndrome) in cocaine users, compared to less than 1% in the general population.

When a woman uses cocaine in the third trimester, it increases the risk of placental abruption tenfold. Significant prematurity and increased growth restrictions have also been documented, as well as genital and urinary malformations and skull defects. In addition, stillbirths have been documented in 8–10% of cocaine users.

While some people might argue that marijuana is not harmful, the vast majority of physicians strongly condemn its use. Because it's an illegal drug, it's difficult to have observational studies of women who have taken it. Although the information is limited, most doctors strongly feel that their patients should *not* take marijuana.

Computers and X-Rays

In general, sitting in front of a computer or a television set is safe. Most of the radiation that modern TVs or computers put out is negligible. The amount of radiation put out from a medical X-ray is also fairly low, but if possible, avoid the use of X-rays in the first trimester. Always let a doctor or dentist know if you are pregnant, so that they can shield your abdomen with a lead apron. If a woman is experiencing a medical or dental condition and an X-ray is recommended to aid in the diagnosis, then she should not hesitate to have it performed as long as the doctor is aware of her condition and can take the necessary precautions.

FROM THE DOCTOR'S PERSPECTIVE...

I once had a dentist call me and say that he refused to take care of an abscess in a woman's mouth because she was pregnant, and he didn't want to X-ray or treat her at all. This is ridiculous, because the danger of the abscess festering and causing serious problems was much worse than the potential damage of an X-ray. I sent this patient to another dentist who didn't have any problem treating her condition.

The Absolute Minimum

There is a small, but very vital person growing inside of you in the first three months of your pregnancy. Take care of that person.

- The first trimester is when all the important organs and organ systems are forming in the baby.
- Anything that you ingest, good or bad, has the potential for harming the baby.
- What can be a bad habit for you can be deadly for the baby growing inside of you.

In This Chapter

- What the heck is "good nutrition?"
- How much weight can I gain (or how much is too much)?
- What do I do about cravings?
- What ramifications are there for being overweight or underweight?

7

Nutrition and Weight Gain

Nutrition—food—the bane and joy of our existence. Gotta have it; don't want to get fat; but with pregnancy there is a built-in excuse to eat (and ergo, gain a few sanctioned pounds.). Or is there? No excuse according to Dr. John, who sees eating a healthful diet as one of the most important things you can do for your baby (and yourself).

FROM THE MOTHER'S PERSPECTIVE...

I must admit that the good doctor and I came to a few blows over this chapter. I was constantly defending the mother's right to eat, while Dr. John kept pre-empting my sage advice with dire consequences to excess weight gain. We finally compromised. I agreed to let him vent and grandstand a bit about not gaining too much weight during pregnancy. He agreed to let me take out his "I'm the doctor; I know best" preachy tone. I'm realistic—it's hard not to gain weight. He's a man—he's never been pregnant and hungry.

Nutrition Affects the Baby Directly

We both recognize that women are sensitive to weight gain and the retention of weight after pregnancy. It's a concern for everyone, and it does affect your long-term health. However, let's face it—you are going to gain some weight while you're pregnant, and if you didn't, the baby would be in danger. The trick is to gain the appropriate amount of weight for the baby's health and yours—it's a balancing act.

As far as pregnancy is concerned, adequate nutrition and weight gain are important because they can affect the baby's health directly. Bad nutrition and improper weight gain (either too much or too little) are both associated with poor perinatal outcomes (translation: the baby's subsequent health can be compromised). For example, excessive weight gain or obesity, poor nutrition or being underweight, and pica (see sidebar) all contribute to poor outcomes for the baby.If you eat a nutritious diet, chances are that your baby will be healthier than if you didn't. The important ingredient (pardon the pun) is to eat foods rich in nutrients (vitamins), rather than foods with empty calories (a perfect example of what not to eat is chips and dip, my personal favorite).

caution

Poor nutrition can affect the development of the fetus's organs and compromise its survival in the first trimester. In the third trimester, inadequate nutrition can affect the baby's growth rate. The third trimester is the most important time for the baby to get its nutrients. If the mother isn't eating properly, the baby will still draw what it needs from the mother, possibly making her anemic or deprived of the necessary nutrients to keep her health intact.

WHAT IS PICA?

Pica is a rare condition that occurs during pregnancy in which the pregnant woman has an unusual urge to eat odd things, most commonly clay or ice. Doctors suspect that the urge might stem from the body having a sense that it needs to improve its iron intake. Although this condition is typically found in third world countries, it has also been documented in the U.S. Keep in mind that nonnutritive substances (not food) can lead to anemia, bowel obstruction (which could require surgical intervention), and nutritional deficiencies. (Moral: Don't eat Play-Dough.)

Defining Good Nutrition and Weight Gain

Good nutrition while you're pregnant isn't vastly different from good nutrition when you aren't pregnant. The operative question being: Was your diet good when you weren't pregnant?

So, while you're pregnant, you should still eat a good variety of fruits, vegetables, proteins, and dairy products, albeit not in excess. The old adage that "you're eating for two" is not accurate information, unfortunately. Rather, you're eating for yourself and a tiny, little microscopic thing inside of you that is infinitesimally small in the beginning. It doesn't even weigh a gram. So, the first three months are not an excuse to gain excess weight!

News flash: You can't eat whatever you want or how much you want. There are still limitations. Generally, the old thinking was that you needed approximately 300 calories per day more than when you weren't pregnant, most of those additional calories coming from proteins. Now, the thinking is that an average-sized woman needs approximately 2200–2500 total calories from the four different food groups.

An average-sized woman, who weighs 135 pounds before the pregnancy (is there anyone out there to whom this applies?), should have an average weight gain of 25–30 pounds during her pregnancy. In a pregnancy lasting 40 weeks, this breaks down to a 5–7 pound weight gain for the first 20 weeks and 1 pound per week for the next 20 weeks. Some of that weight is actually baby weight (that is, it goes to the development of the fetus), but much of it can be attributed to amniotic fluid, the uterus, increased blood volume, and adipose tissue (or fat). Table 7.1 breaks down pretty succinctly where the weight goes.

Table 7.1 Average Breakdown of Weight Gained (lbs) During Pregnancy

Where It Goes...	Weight in Pounds
Baby	5-7
Placenta	1-2
Amniotic Fluid	5-6
Blood Volume	4-5
Uterus	2-3
Breasts	2-3
Fat Stores	7-8
Total	26-34

After you have the baby, you should lose the weight of the baby plus another 4 or 5 pounds, which is approximately 12 pounds. That will give you an additional 12–16 pounds to lose after the baby's birth. And that is the killer weight to lose, in my opinion. If you're nursing, they say it comes off faster (and it does), but you still have to count calories and exercise to get rid of that "baby weight."

Good Foods to Eat

The food pyramid (see Figure 7.1) will give you some general guidelines about the food groups that you should include and portions; however, it has come under some controversy recently (see sidebar).

caution

The jury is still out on how nutritious it is to follow the Atkins or South Beach diets, and now is not the time to try either one of them when you have a baby to worry about. Stay away from dieting!

THE "BUSTED" FOOD PYRAMID

The standard food pyramid that most of us have used over the past few decades is currently being reviewed by the Department of Agriculture because agricultural officials say new research has indicated that the proportions of the food groups may need to be altered to optimize them. Health leaders think that the pyramid can be confusing, and the fact that 60% of Americans are overweight indicates that it is not working. Upshot: It may stay as is; it may change; who knows?

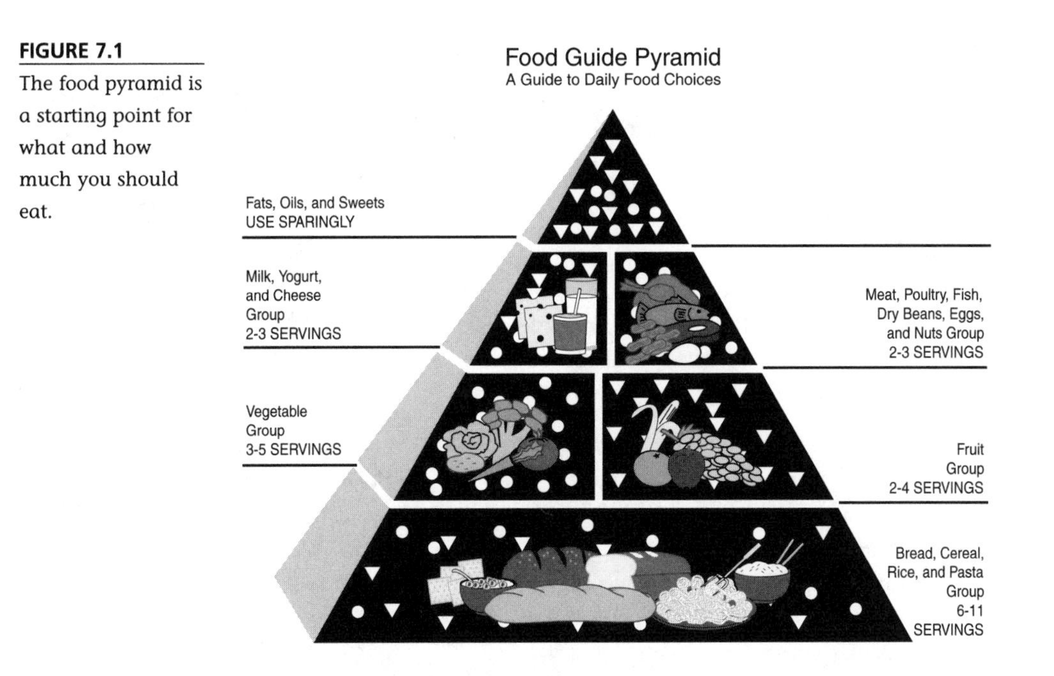

FIGURE 7.1
The food pyramid is a starting point for what and how much you should eat.

Generally, try to follow a basic food plan, allowing for the following food groups on a daily basis:

- Plenty of fruits (at least four servings—look for fruits rich in vitamin C, like oranges, blueberries, and so on)
- Vegetables (at least four or five servings—rich-colored fruits and vegetables are the best, such as broccoli, spinach, tomatoes, roots, and so forth)
- Legumes (beans and peas) and nuts (make sure you aren't allergic to nuts first)
- Dairy foods (either a quart of milk or two–three servings of other dairy products)
- Lean meats (red meats are a great source of iron) or fish (low-mercury fish) and protein (at least three servings)
- Whole grain cereals and breads
- Some fats and oils (olive oil is a good heart-healthy oil or sunflower or safflower oil—monosaturated oils are better than polysaturated, such as vegetable oil)
- Eight glasses of water a day (or more)

Try to limit or avoid the following foods in your daily diet:

- Limit empty calories found in snacks, such as any kind of chips.
- Limit salt intake.
- Limit sugar intake.
- Avoid soft cheeses, such as feta, Brie, Camembert, etc. (avoid all unpasteurized products because they might have some bacteria present).
- Avoid cold cuts from deli counters (not only are they processed foods with extra salt, but they could contain harmful bacteria).
- Limit regular soft drinks to one per day (filled with extra calories, high fructose corn syrup contributes to obesity).
- Diet sodas are generally OK, but don't overindulge. Make sure that you're not an individual who has a problem with PKU (Phenylketonurics), although this would not apply to most individuals.
- Avoid caffeine if possible or limit it (as it could be harmful and cause birth defects in the baby).
- Use caution with fresh water fish (as they could be contaminated with pesticides and carcinogens).
- Use caution with fresh tuna, swordfish, or shark (could be exposed to mercury poisoning—see sidebar).
- Always avoid alcohol (as it could cause fetal alcohol syndrome). There is no safe amount of alcohol you can drink during pregnancy.

caution

If you have swelling, the natural reaction is to cut back on fluids or water intake. Don't do this! In a healthy woman, the excess water does not go to swelling; it goes out in the form of free urine (as opposed to the paying kind). Swelling is a different mechanism. Always, always drink your water—as much as possible. And consider cutting back on your salt intake. Unless you're cooking everything from scratch at home, take the saltshaker off the dinner table. Your food is probably already loaded with salt without adding any more.

note

There are limited studies about how safe Aspartame (an artificial sweetener) is in pregnancy, but to date there has been no legitimate concern raised with this product and fetal development.

THE SCOOP ABOUT FISH

Basically, what we're concerned about here is the level of mercury found in cold-water fish, for example, tuna, swordfish, and shark. The concern is that the level of mercury that was previously thought to be present in these fish was sufficiently low to negate any adverse effects on the pregnant woman and her unborn child. However, recent evidence suggests that the mercury levels may be much higher than originally perceived. Mercury can be hazardous to the development of a fetus. This issue is undergoing extensive scrutiny at the present time. While pregnant women do not have to avoid these products entirely, they should still eat them with caution and consult with their doctor. After all, tuna is an excellent source of protein, and is generally a healthful food; however, these issues do raise some concerns.

Nitty Gritty Details (Some Don'ts—Forget the "Do's")

Dr. John says that women don't like to eat the same things that guys like; for example, they don't go overboard on hot dogs and hamburgers. (Sometimes, I wonder what planet this man came from. I can inhale those items with the best of them.) As far as his experience goes, his patients tend to have a "sweet spot" for the sweets (ergo, pastries, ice cream, cakes, cookies). His patients may deny that they eat fried foods, but when it comes to asking them about sweets, they get a guilty, sly grin on their faces and Dr. John swears that they act as if he's been looking over their shoulders, the guilt is so obvious.

Dr. John's advice: Don't eliminate sweets, but limit their consumption to once a week. (This man is oh, so NOT realistic!)

Another "Don't": Be careful about your salt intake. Usually, there is more than enough salt in processed food, so you can throw away your saltshaker, or at least remove it from the table. Excess salt will increase your swelling, particularly of the extremities (legs and hands). And trust me, it isn't worth the pain. Swelling can also affect your blood pressure, causing it to increase and making it more difficult for you to walk (not a good thing).

THOSE PESKY CRAVINGS AND AVERSIONS

Ice cream, pickles, peanut butter on bread with butter or mayo...whatever your craving is, it's sure to come in the middle of the night when you least expect it, but most want to honor it. Generally, cravings are harmless, so indulge them if they aren't too far out of the norm. Obviously, don't eat anything that will make you sick. (If it makes your partner sick to watch you eat whatever abomination you've concocted, then have him leave the room.)

Some women experience cravings all the way through their pregnancy, but most find that the first trimester is the worst. Blame it on hormones, because that is probably what is causing it.

Food aversions are equally puzzling. You might find some foods that you used to adore, but that are suddenly making you sick now. If so, avoid them. It's the body's way of telling you that you can't tolerate something. Chances are good that your food preferences will adjust back to normal after the baby is born.

What to Eat if You're Nauseous

If you're nauseous, have morning sickness, or simply don't feel like eating, you may start to lose more weight than you should. In this case, be sure to drink more fluids than usual, as you don't want to become dehydrated. If you feel faint, call your doctor for a checkup.

Do try to eat something. Start with smaller portions of food and stick to light foods, such as soups, crackers, graham crackers, gelatin (Jello), Seven Up, or anything that appeals to you that you think you can keep down. Eat smaller meals more often. Try eating at different times of the day. Perhaps the morning is a bad time for you, but your stomach feels more settled in the afternoon. In this case, eat in the afternoon. If you are unable to eat after trying these remedies, call your care provider for instructions.

HEARTBURN

If you have heartburn, avoid spicy and acidic foods. Don't eat late at night and don't lie down immediately after you eat. Try to allow more time for digestion. Always check with your doctor before taking any medications, in this case, antacids.

For Those Who Are Overweight or Underweight

Although all of us would like to start our pregnancy in the best possible shape ever, it doesn't always happen that way. At the time of conception, you may be either underweight or overweight, and either condition could cause serious problems for your pregnancy.

If You're Underweight

Believe it or not, being severely underweight is as much of a problem as being overweight. If a woman weighs under, say 100 pounds, then doctors will probably want her to gain more weight than the average-sized woman, possibly gaining 30–40 pounds instead of 25. The point is for the baby to get what it needs from the mother. In an underweight woman, the task of the doctor is to find out why the mother is underweight. Some typical causes might be that she's not taking care of herself, she has an eating disorder, and she smokes, uses drugs, or has any number of conditions. Any of these causes poses a serious risk to the baby's health and needs to be addressed immediately.

For those women who are simply small-boned or normally very thin, the doctor will probably put you in touch with a nutritionist to make sure that you're getting the proper amount of nutrition for both you and the baby.

FROM THE DOCTOR'S PERSPECTIVE...

When a woman is pregnant, the basic principle for all doctors is that they are taking care of two patients, not just one. A balanced diet will give the mother all she needs during pregnancy, as well as addressing the dietary needs of the baby growing inside of her.

Most doctors try to be sensitive to weight issues, but we don't want to say a woman's eating habits are OK when they're not. Although most women won't change their eating habits significantly when they're pregnant, we still try to educate them. We don't want to risk the baby's health. Sometimes, just giving a woman little tips helps, like don't take the escalator, take the stairs; or don't drink too many fruit juices, because the nutritional benefit is quickly outweighed by the excess calories; or park far away at the grocery store; don't take the spot that is close.

Remember that your doctor has your best interests (and your baby's) at heart. Work with your doctors—they are not the enemy, but your supporter.

If You're Overweight

If you start off your pregnancy overweight (which will be defined by your doctor), then your doctor might restrict your weight gain during pregnancy to 15–20 pounds, which figures to a gain of 1/2 pound per week. In this case the mother doesn't necessarily need extra nutrition, but needs to eat healthy, normal portions of food. Pregnancy works like a kind of parasite on the mother's body, taking what it needs from the mother. The overweight woman probably doesn't have a problem with her nutrition, per se, unless she is deriving all her calories from poor nutritional sources. The baby needs good substrates (or basic building blocks) for development.

Some problems that overweight women might face in pregnancy include:

- High blood pressure
- Diabetes
- Increased risk for cesarean section
- Higher risk for shoulder dystocia during a vaginal delivery (where the shoulder of the baby gets stuck or impacted behind the mother's pubic bone)
- Operative or c-section complications
- Greater back pain or limited mobility
- More weight to lose after birth

tip

The trend now is to individualize eating plans for pregnant women by having either the doctor or a nutritionist calculate a woman's BMI (body mass index) and recommend a personal diet plan for each individual. Then the doctor will track your weight gain or loss during your pregnancy and make appropriate recommendations for correcting any problems that might arise (see the BMI figures in Chapter 5).

Vitamins

If a woman is eating a balanced nutritious diet, usually that diet will provide all the vitamins needed during pregnancy. Unfortunately, achieving a balanced diet poses a challenge for many women. Fortunately, though, vitamin supplementation in the form of prenatal vitamins is appropriate to address some of these deficiencies in a diet. Dr. John thinks it's a good idea, and he almost always recommends vitamins for his patients.

Prenatal vitamins will contain the necessary iron as well as other nutrients that a pregnant and lactating woman will require. However, occasionally additional iron supplementation is prescribed for a woman who still has an iron deficiency demonstrated by a third trimester blood test. At that time, additional iron may be prescribed after you have the results of your test.

Some women have difficulty taking prenatal vitamins because they make them feel nauseous or sick. There are alternatives. For example, you may have better luck with another brand of vitamin with a different formulation. If you still have difficulty, then the doctor may recommend that you take a Flintstones children's vitamin (no kidding!).

tip

If you take iron or a multivitamin with orange juice, the vitamin C in the OJ will help your body absorb the iron more efficiently.

Folic acid is another important ingredient in a woman's diet. Folic acid is recommended during pregnancy (and often if a woman is trying to get pregnant) because the risk of having a neural tube defect in your baby is decreased substantially. A neural tube defect could manifest as spina bifida or the absence of a brain. Generally, it occurs in 1 out of 1500 births in the U.S. With 4 million births per year, the individual's risk may be low, but the population, in general, is higher. This defect occurs more frequently in geographical areas of the country where nutrition isn't as good as it should be.

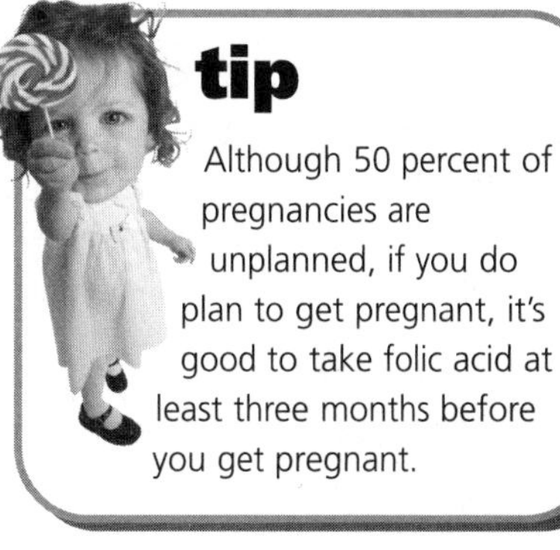

tip

Although 50 percent of pregnancies are unplanned, if you do plan to get pregnant, it's good to take folic acid at least three months before you get pregnant.

The recommended dosage of folic acid is approximately 400 micrograms a day, which is exactly what is included in prenatal vitamins. Fortunately, folic acid is incorporated in many foods that are commercially available, like cereals, as well as prenatal vitamins.

In rare cases, if a woman has had a baby previously with one of these defects, the doctor will probably recommend that you take 4 milligrams a day (a larger dosage) to reduce the chances of future babies having this defect.

FROM THE DOCTOR'S PERSPECTIVE...

For some women who are reading this book, a financial difficulty or the inability to get to a grocery store may keep them from getting adequate nutrition, so there is a federal supplemental food program for women and infant children (called WIC) that could be helpful in these situations. Your local hospital or local county health department can direct you to the right place, or you can call information to get a phone number. Usually, WIC will give you a form to take to your doctor. Then the doctor will authenticate your pregnancy, and WIC will give you food, products, or resources that you need in order to sustain a healthy pregnancy. This program is also helpful after the baby is born. Don't be ashamed to call them. Everyone needs help sometimes, and you don't want to risk your baby's life or your own.

THE ABSOLUTE MINIMUM

- Pregnancy is not an excuse to blimp out.
- What you eat directly affects your health and your baby's well being.
- Take your prenatal vitamins religiously. A small amount of prevention is well worth the cure.

In This Chapter

- Can you exercise when you're pregnant?
- What types of exercises are good for you?
- Can exercise be dangerous when you're pregnant?
- What about having sex?

8

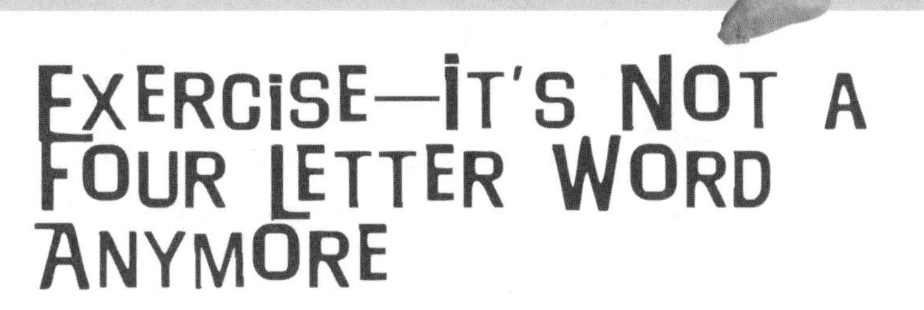

Exercise—It's Not a Four Letter Word Anymore

When it comes to exercise, as Nike says, "Just do it!" Years ago, doctors often cautioned pregnant women against exercise, fearing that it could precipitate labor or endanger their pregnancy. Today's physicians are more enlightened and have discovered that exercising during pregnancy has many short-term and long-term benefits for both mother and baby.

The Unwritten Rules

In general, the rule of thumb is to use common sense when it comes to following an exercise regimen during pregnancy. First, make sure that you are in good physical health and that your doctor does *not* prohibit or limit your exercise for any reason (always check with a doctor first). Second, don't take up a new strenuous physical activity now that you're pregnant—for example, something that you've never done in the past. This is *not* the time to start new physical activities. Third, don't do anything that you have doubts about or lack the confidence in your ability to complete in a safe manner. Always, always consider safety first. Stay away from exercises that present risks to the abdomen.

THE NO-EXERCISE EXERCISE

Kegel exercises were named after Dr. Kegel who originally described the muscle group that aids in controlling urine outflow (also known as the pubococcygeous muscle or pc muscle—not politically correct, however). The exercises are simple to do. Next time you're urinating, use the muscles to practice stopping your urine midstream. By strengthening these muscles, you may have better control over your urine outflow. So what's the big deal? Why do it? Because some scientists feel that pregnancy weakens these muscles so that later on a woman has urinary incontinence. Scientists and doctors debate whether it is pregnancy itself that affects the PC or the labor and delivery of a vaginal birth that contributes to weakening these muscles. In truth, it's probably a little of both. Although it's unclear how much this exercise helps during pregnancy, it's clear that it doesn't hurt. You can practice tightening the muscle group and holding it 10 20 seconds, as often as you like, and the beauty of it is that no one knows you're doing it (you won't even break a sweat).

What's Good for You

Walk, walk, walk, and then walk some more. Walking is one of the best exercises for increasing blood flow and burning calories. Running and jogging are OK if you are used to them. Riding bikes is a safe exercise, presuming you're stable on the bike and don't fall off. Swimming is a great cardio-vascular exercise that supports the stomach, as well as the joints. No diving, please. It's preferable to swim in a clean, well-kept, chlorinated pool, rather than a lake or an ocean where infection might be a concern. Low impact aerobics are excellent, as is yoga for pregnancy or regular yoga (see Figure 8.1). Make sure the instructor or any trainer of an exercise regimen knows that you are pregnant, so the exercises can be tailored to your condition.

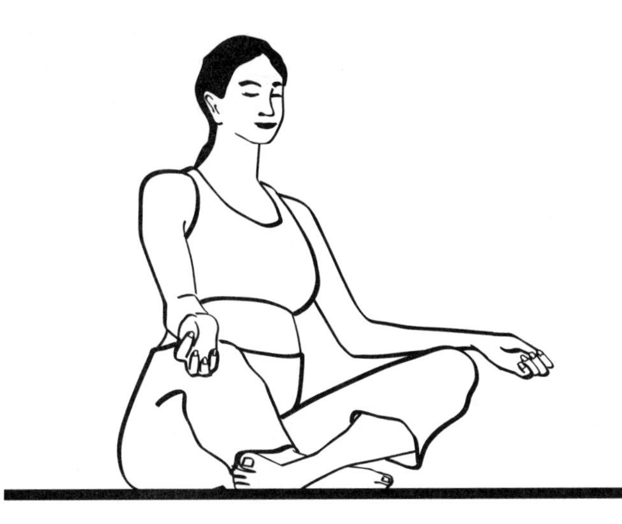

FIGURE 8.1
Besides the obvious physical benefits of stretching with yoga, you will also benefit from the breathing and relaxation techniques.

FOR THE WORKING MOM

It's definitely more difficult for the working mother to work in (pun intended) exercise; however, it is not impossible. First, take the stairs instead of the elevator whenever possible. Second, walk on your breaks—a short walk is better than no walk at all. Also, try walking or working out on your lunch hour. Sometimes, workplaces will have a gym where you can get some treadmill or bike time in. If not, take 20 minutes at home after work to devote to some cardiovascular exercise (walk around the block). Also, do stretches at work, including your Kegel exercises. No one will be the wiser, except you. Prop your feet up occasionally and take time to get up and move around, not staying in one position for too long.

Don't forget that weekends count. If you can get in three days a week of 20 minutes of exercise (get that heart rate up!), that's better than none at all. Of course, more is always better.

What Isn't Good

Stay away from anything that could do harm to your abdomen, cause you to fall, or hurt you in any way. While many women do ride horses during pregnancy, it is considered risky, due to the possibility of a fall. Absolutely no cross-country riding or jumping should be allowed in the latter stages of pregnancy, and it could be damaging in the earlier stages as well. Most physicians would have no problem with an easy loping pace on a horse, but strenuous galloping should be avoided. Riding a motorcycle cross-country would not be the best sport while pregnant. This is not the time to run a marathon or participate in any regular strenuous exercises. Team sports are permissible, depending on the risk of injury. Basketball could be dangerous if you are knocked over or elbowed in the abdomen. Tennis should be fine, as long as you don't let the ball hit you in the stomach.

POTENTIAL RISKS TO THE ABDOMEN

Be careful in a weight room. It's OK to continue lifting free weights or a lifting bar, but you might want to decrease the weight. You absolutely *don't* want to drop the bar or weights on your stomach, so it might be better to discontinue this type of exercise altogether. Be aware that your center of gravity will change the farther along you get into the pregnancy. Even Nautilus machines have the potential to injure you if you pull incorrectly or a weight drops unexpectedly.

caution

Jacuzzis and hot tubs are more risky in the first trimester because of the high temperatures involved. Any extreme temperature variation (too hot or too cold) may have adverse effects on the fetus or may cause fetal anomalies. Unfortunately, doctors don't understand the mechanism by which the anomalies occur, since there are very few studies designed to look at this concern, for obvious reasons. The concern in earlier studies was that extreme temperatures could lead to limb defects, for example, an arm or a leg not growing properly.

The Benefits of Exercise

Women who exercise usually have a better pregnancy, in terms of being more comfortable physically and healthier for the duration of the pregnancy and afterwards. Often, they tolerate the stress and pain of labor better and sometimes they don't require as many meds during labor, or can even get away with taking no meds at all. Stretching exercises can be particularly useful for later ease in labor and delivery (see Figure 8.2).

With regular exercise during pregnancy, women also recuperate faster after the birth of the baby, whether they have a vaginal delivery or a C-section. Obviously, an additional benefit is not gaining as much weight during pregnancy. In general, exercising seems to go along with eating better and maintaining a more positive attitude toward the pregnancy. Since exercising releases endorphins, it also helps with emotional stress and potential depression.

FROM THE DOCTOR'S PERSPECTIVE...

Doctors know that exercise is truly beneficial for pregnant women. Many colleagues of mine (obviously females) make sure to follow an exercise regimen throughout their pregnancy. I once had a woman who exercised right up to her delivery. This woman came in to the hospital to get checked because she thought she might be in pre-labor (she'd had children before). Surprisingly, she was 8 centimeters dilated, and wasn't feeling too bad. She'd come straight to the hospital after pushing a lawnmower and mowing her entire lawn. Her labor only took an hour and a half, and she recovered quickly.

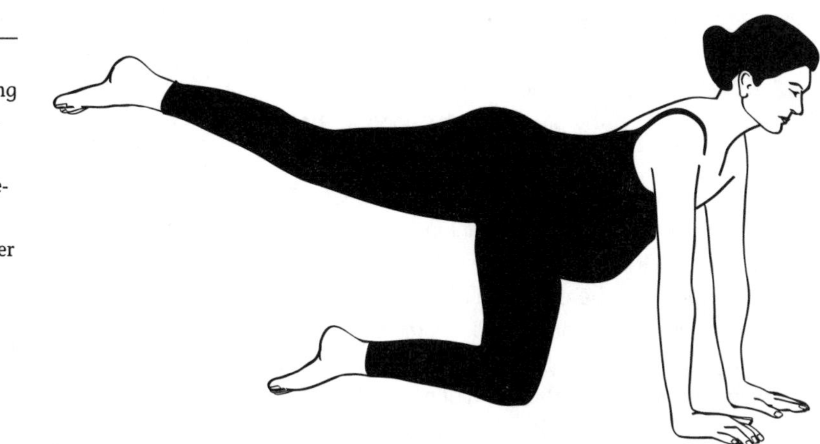

FIGURE 8.2
Stretching is beneficial during and after pregnancy, but has the added benefit of making you more limber during labor and delivery.

A Checklist Before Exercising

So, you've decided to exercise. Here are a few simple, but important, rules to follow.

- ✓ Drink lots of water. Carry along a bottle of water or a sports drink with you.
- ✓ Wear loose, comfortable clothing (don't get too hot or too cold).
- ✓ Wear comfortable shoes that fit well. (Remember, your feet may tend to swell from fluid retention.)
- ✓ Do some stretching exercises in advance to get your muscles warmed up and flexible before starting your exercise regimen.
- ✓ Be aware of your center of gravity as it changes. As pregnancy continues, the center of gravity shifts forward, so women lean backward to compensate. As the shoulders move back and the lower back protrudes forward, accentuating the curvature of the lower spine, the unnatural position can lead to strain on the back muscles and cause back pain. It can also cause you to be a bit off-balance and less coordinated than usual.
- ✓ Get plenty of rest. Don't exercise if you're too tired.

note

Hormonal changes can also cause back pain. The hormone relaxin loosens the pelvic ligaments in order to accommodate the growing pregnancy and labor.

GET DRUNK ON PERSPECTIVE...

Most people walk around in a mildly dehydrated state, even when they are not pregnant. It's kind of dumb, because we feel better when we are adequately hydrated. A pregnant woman should strive for at least 8–10 glasses of water a day, which does not include soda, coffee, tea, or milk. Those beverages are extra after the water consumption. Try to drink as much water as possible during the pregnancy. It's good for both mother and baby.

Why water? Water helps with the blood flow, and it improves uterine profusion, meaning that it optimizes blood flow to the uterus. The benefits: the baby gets more oxygen and the exchange of waste and nutrients between mother and baby becomes more efficient. Insuring adequate water intake can contribute toward having a normal amount of amniotic fluid around the baby. The amniotic fluid keeps the baby floating and keeps the umbilical cord from being compressed. With a lower amount of amniotic fluid, there is more of a risk of the baby sitting on the cord and compressing it in the later stages of pregnancy. Unfortunately, you might not know this until you perceived less movement in the baby.

So...drink up! You can't hurt yourself by drinking too much water as long as your diet is well balanced.

note

Pre-eclampsia is the development of high blood pressure with protein in the urine and generally occurs in the second half of gestation (after 20 weeks). If it goes untreated, it can be extremely dangerous for the mother, sometimes resulting in seizures.

Pre-term labor is defined as a pregnancy that goes into labor at less than 36 weeks gestation. Pre-term labor means that regular uterine contractions occur along with a cervical dilation. In other words, the baby might be born prematurely because you've started into labor early.

Don't confuse pre-term labor with Braxton Hicks contractions. These contractions (feel like a tightening of the uterus) can mimic real contractions. The difference is that they don't occur at regular intervals, and the cervix isn't dilated.

If you are diabetic or have gestational diabetes (related to pregnancy), it is good to be physically active.

When *Not* to Exercise

There are some definite conditions during pregnancy where exercise should be avoided at all costs. If you have pre-eclampsia or pre-term labor, your doctor will *not* let you exercise.

If you have pain, spotting, bleeding, or have an unusual discharge, do not exercise.

If you're feeling light-headed, don't exercise. Pregnant women have a higher tendency to feel light-headed due to changes in blood volume and blood pressure and how the blood vessels constrict and dilate during pregnancy. This normal condition can lead to dizziness if a woman gets up too fast or lies flat on her back (particularly during the second half of the second trimester). If you are light-headed, it could also be from dehydration. Take a break and drink some water or a sports drink.

Exercise While Traveling

Traveling naturally precludes exercising or moving around a whole lot, which can be dangerous for pregnant women. Make sure you get an aisle seat, so you can get up and move around easily. Women who are pregnant have a higher predisposition to forming blood clots in their legs, so movement of the legs is imperative. You should walk at least 10 minutes out of every hour on a flight.

It's wise to drink a liter of a sports drink before boarding the plane (in other words, tank up); then continue to drink water while flying because there is a tendency to get dehydrated while flying. Hydrate, hydrate, hydrate (i.e., drink, drink, drink). Of course, that aisle seat will be a necessity if you do—and you'll get your exercise naturally by marching back and forth to the bathroom.

The Ultimate Exercise—Sex! (or Sex—It's Still a Three-Letter Word)

Depending on your feelings about the matter (and your partner's), sex can be a fun (three letters) and natural type of exercise, particularly if your partner is amenable. In most cases, your sex life should not be curtailed in any way, barring unforeseen circumstances like morning sickness interfering. (It's not particularly sexy or flattering to upchuck while your partner is being amorous.) Occasionally, a woman will feel less like having sex because she's tired or not feeling well; however, just as frequently, a woman may have an increased libido—always good for her mate.

When to Have Sex

It's important for your marriage/relationship that you still make time for sex, even though you're pregnant. Again, to quote Nike—just do it! Otherwise, there is the risk that your husband might get jealous of the baby before it's even born or feel as if he's coming second in your life. It sounds immature, but it happens. Although you may feel like hibernating for a few months, your husband is still very much alive and needs your attention. Schedule dates and time alone. It will pay off in good feelings all-round.

An FYI: The baby does *not* know you're having sex; nor does he/she care, so don't worry about a "third person" watching you.

FROM THE DOCTOR'S PERSPECTIVE...
Some doctors suggest that a woman who is at full term and ready to deliver should use sex to stimulate labor. Marta insists that it's an ancient tribal custom, although I've never heard that theory.

FROM THE PATIENT'S PERSPECTIVE...
Sorry, but when I was ready to deliver, sex was the last thing on my mind. Ancient tribal customs aside (and I have heard it somewhere, Dr. John!), anyone who tried to touch me that way might not have lived to tell about it. A woman near labor is not a pretty thing to behold or be around (at least not in my case).

When *Not* to Have Sex

Use common sense about not having sex. If intercourse causes you pain, stop it and consult with your doctor as soon as possible. If you have any unusual discharge before, during, or after sex; or if you have a leakage of fluid, these are conditions to report to your doctor. If you're bleeding, and it is undiagnosed bleeding, it needs to be checked out immediately. If you're having any kind of uterine contractions that you're unsure about, it's probably *not* a good time to have sex, and you should report your condition to your doctor.

Always be careful that your partner does not hurt you in any way, particularly your abdomen. Prolonged direct compression of a woman's abdomen during intercourse (the missionary position) could be harmful for obvious reasons (particularly in the later stages of pregnancy), but most other positions are OK. If your back hurts, you can always prop pillows under it or do whatever it takes to get comfortable.

In most cases, physicians will recommend that you should not have sex if you're in pre-term labor, for fear that you might stimulate the labor. Also, if you have placenta previa, it is generally advisable not to have intercourse or put anything in the vagina (you don't want anything to have contact with the cervix). Of course, if your water breaks, skip sex and go straight to the hospital (do not pass go; do not collect $200).

It's probably alright to have oral sex, but doctors don't know for sure. Orgasm in a woman can cause contractions of the uterus. It's unclear what component of sex may contribute to increased uterine contractions that could lead to pre-term labor. Doctors don't know if it's related to chemical reactions or a prostaglandin release. In other words, is it the physical act of intercourse that stimulates the contractions or is it caused by a woman's orgasm? These questions are difficult to answer, since the data is limited, but this is the reason that most physicians still suggest pelvic rest (or no sex) if a woman is in pre-term labor.

The Absolute Minimum

If you can exercise comfortably and without pain, then get out there and move. Exercising will keep you in shape during the pregnancy and probably make your labor and delivery easier and more efficient.

- Exercise responsibly, meaning don't do anything that causes you pain at the time or later.
- Walking is probably the best exercise during pregnancy. Buy a pedometer and track your progress.
- Carry a water bottle with you at all times and use it. Getting dehydrated is one of the worst things you can do to your body. Staying hydrated is one of the best.
- Feel good about yourself and enjoy sex. You're still a desirable woman, and your husband will appreciate the attention.
- Having a baby does not mean limiting your life; it means expanding it, so keep doing the things you were doing before you were pregnant (within reason).

IN THIS CHAPTER

- What are the normal tests you should expect to be given?
- What do these tests mean?
- Are there any optional tests that might be useful?
- When do doctors order the high-risk tests?

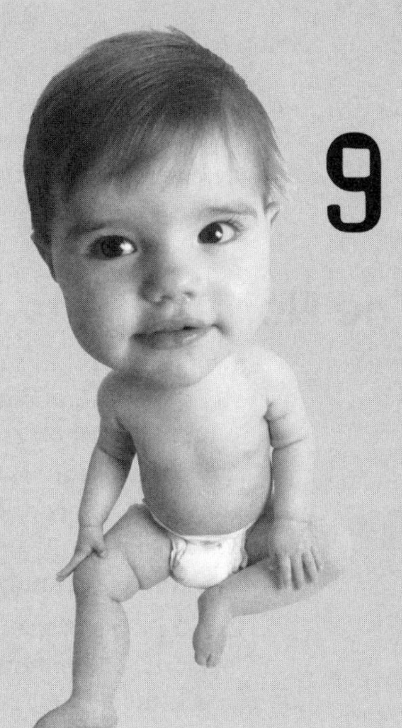

9

TESTS PERFORMED DURING PREGNANCY

We wrote this chapter mostly as a reference chapter and because I wanted you to know more about all those tests you take when you're pregnant, most of which are Greek to all patients. So, Dr. John cheerfully obliged in explaining the ins and outs of the tests you're likely to receive (and some you won't). We structured the chapter so that you can easily look up the test and then find out why doctors consider it to be important.

You'll find two types of tests performed during your pregnancy: those that are considered routine and that everyone receives and those that are done for patients who are considered to be at risk.

The Normal Tests

In your first visit, the physician will do a thorough gynecological exam. Your cervix will be checked, and a clinical pelvimetry exam performed, where the doctor uses his hands to get an estimate of the size of the pelvic bones to determine if your anatomy is adequate for delivering a baby vaginally. Other areas to be checked will be the breasts, heart, and lungs. The doctor probably won't recheck the cervix again until it is medically indicated, for example, if there is a concern for preterm labor or if a woman is actually in labor.

Here are some of the more common tests that will be performed on *most* women. Obviously, all the tests that are ordered are up to your physician, so if you don't get a specific test, don't panic. Your doctor may not think it is necessary for you to have that particular one.

CBC

One of the first tests that you'll receive is a CBC (complete blood count). This test checks your hematocrit and hemoglobin, as well as platelet count. Translation for laypeople like us: Hemoglobin and hematocrit measure your potential for anemia (see Figure 9.1).

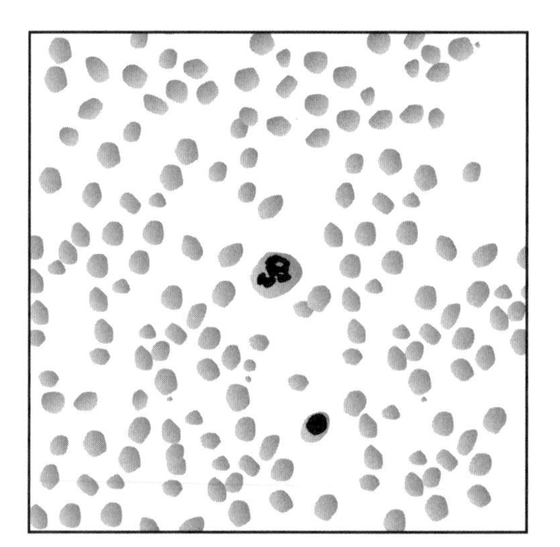

FIGURE 9.1
A blood smear gives your physician valuable information about your pregnancy.

Why it's important (hematocrit and hemoglobin): Those women who are anemic need to be identified well ahead of delivery so that therapy can improve their low blood count. Physiologic anemia can be problematic to the patient, as discussed earlier in Chapter 5.

Why it's important (platelet count): Because a woman will lose half a liter of blood on average at delivery. The platelet count measures the blood's ability to clot. With a low platelet count, a patient is at risk for bleeding to death.

note

At the beginning of the third trimester, some tests are repeated, such as a CBC to monitor for potential anemia that could occur later in the pregnancy. The reason for a CBC in the third trimester is pretty much confined to the anemia issue as far as the blood test is concerned.

Approximately 5% of pregnant women have *asymptomatic* UTI, which means they have no discernible symptoms to tip off them or their doctor to the fact that they might have an infection (ergo, the need for the test).

Urine Screen

A urine screen is primarily performed to check for urinary tract infections (no surprise there), more commonly known as *UTIs*. Occasionally, the urine screen may pick up other abnormalities of renal function, such as excess sugar or protein. Pregnant women seem to be more prone to UTIs than they are normally. If the screening tests positive for an infection, often the doctor will order a culture to determine which organisms are responsible for the infection. That way the doctor can determine antibiotic sensitivity, finding out which antibiotic would be most effective against a specific organism.

Why it's important: Because UTIs can lead to kidney infections. If the infection is allowed to progress, this could lead to harmful effects on the pregnancy, as well as increase the risk for sepsis (a serious life-threatening infection involving the blood) in the mother.

Blood Type and Rh Status and Antibody Screen

Blood tests will check your blood type, your Rh status, and an antibody screen. Your blood type needs to be checked so that a potential mix-up of bloods can be averted if there is a need for a transfusion. Rh negative women need to be identified in advance so that they can be considered as candidates for RhoGAM, an immunoglobulin that is given at 28 weeks of pregnancy and within 72 hours of delivery in order for the mother to keep from becoming Rh sensitized. Occasionally, RhoGAM is also given when there is a potential risk for fetal blood to mix with the mother's blood, such as in a car accident or in amniocentesis.

WHY IS THE RH FACTOR IMPORTANT?

The concern for knowing the mother's Rh type centers on the medical concept called *isoimmunization*. Isoimmunization refers to the development of antibodies to red blood cell markers following exposure to such markers from another individual. In pregnancy, the other individual is the fetus, which contains 50% of its genetic material contributed from the father. If the pregnant mother is exposed to fetal blood cells during pregnancy or delivery, she has the potential to develop antibodies to fetal red blood cells. This condition can occur in the current pregnancy or more likely in a future pregnancy. These antibodies could cross the placenta and attack the fetus's blood cells, which could, in turn, cause anemia of the fetus and potential death.

The percentage of Rh negative pregnant women married to Rh positive men who will be isoimmunized is approximately 5%. Because 75% of all women have evidence of fetal maternal hemorrhaging after delivery (mixing of their own blood and the infant's blood), there exists a high potential for mixing of the two bloods.

note

RhoGAM is Rh immunoglobulin prepared from patients previously sensitive to RhD. RhoGAM absorbs the positive fetal Rh blood cell markers and blocks the formation of maternal Rh antibodies at the time of exposure, which usually occurs at delivery. All women who have never been sensitized to Rh positive blood should receive RhoGAM within 72 hours of delivery. With the current practice recommendations, the risk of subsequent sensitization decreases from 15% to 2% (this statistic is valid if you just gave RhoGAM within 72 hours of having a baby). If you also give RhoGAM at 28 weeks or the beginning of the third trimester, in addition to giving it postpartum, then the risk is reduced to 0.2%.

Why it's important (RhoGAM): Giving this medication prevents the mother's body from mounting an antibody response against an Rh positive baby in future pregnancies.

An antibody screen detects antibodies, both Rh and less common types, that may occur in the fetus or newborn.

Why it's important (antibody screen): Antibodies have the potential for causing blood disease in the fetus and newborn.

Syphilis Screen

Although syphilis is more common in urban areas of the U.S., it can be found anywhere. If a syphilis test comes back positive, then an FTA (Free Treponemal Antibody) test is performed. If this test is positive, then syphilis is officially diagnosed.

When a woman is pregnant, the only medicine she can take for syphilis is penicillin. If she weren't pregnant, she could be treated with other medications.

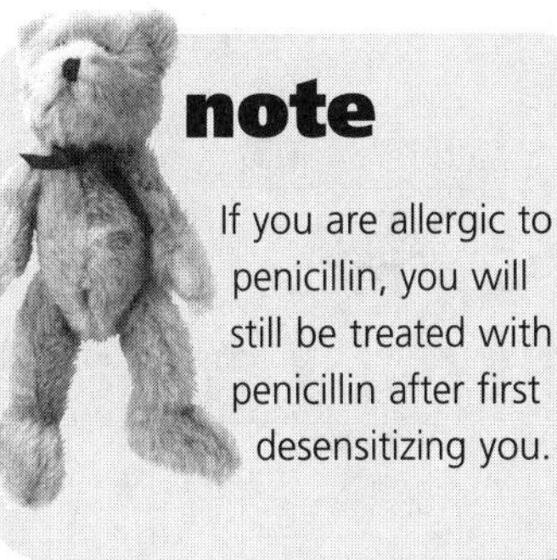

note

If you are allergic to penicillin, you will still be treated with penicillin after first desensitizing you.

Why it's important: Syphilis can lead to preterm labor or even death. Syphilis can also affect the baby's growth and cause congenital anomalies. In the early part of the 20th century (1900s), 40% of all baby's deaths were related to syphilis, but in recent times syphilis has rarely been identified as a cause of death. However, because of the increase in syphilis in the U.S., increased surveillance is recommended. In the past decade alone, maternal and congenital syphilis has increased several fold in the U.S. The infection can occur during any trimester of pregnancy. Overall, untreated syphilis can be transmitted to the fetus or embryo in at least 50% of all pregnancies, causing serious problems with the baby, not the least of which is death.

Rubella Screen

Due to the increased vaccination process of the past 25 years, rubella syndrome is now rare in the U.S.; however, approximately 10% of pregnant women may be susceptible to it (meaning they have no evidence of antibodies for it). If a screen test shows that you are not immune to rubella (in other words that you can contract it), then the hospital will immunize you after your baby is born. You can't be immunized while you're pregnant because it's a live-borne virus so the baby could be affected. If you know you are susceptible to rubella, you should limit your exposure to high-risk sources, such as children who might contract it. Definitely stay far away from anyone you know who has an outbreak of the virus.

caution

Even if you had an MMR (measles, mumps, rubella) shot when you were a kid, it might not be effective anymore. Rubella is more commonly known as a type of measles.

Why it's important: If a woman gets the infection while pregnant, she could transmit the virus to her baby. The virus could increase the baby's risk of congenital anomalies, preterm labor issues, and severe medical complications.

Hepatitis B

Women who have hepatitis B or have been infected previously can transmit the disease to their infant during or after birth, so it's important to discuss in advance what the best way to deliver your baby should be.

Why it's important: Babies can become carriers and develop chronic hepatitis. Between 25–35% of those people infected eventually die from cirrhosis or liver cancer.

Pap Smear

A pap smear will be done if you haven't had one already in the previous year. Doctors are looking for precancerous changes in the cervix. If necessary, they might perform a colposcopy and a cervix biopsy for further diagnosis. They will also check for chlamydia and gonorrhea through a culture from the vagina. The treatment for both chlamydia and gonorrhea is antibiotics.

Why it's important (gonorrhea): Gonorrhea can cause potential blindness in a newborn. It can also cause chorioamnionitis, which is an infection of the membrane surrounding the bag of water that surrounds the baby. After the bag of water is ruptured, there is a higher incidence of premature births and subsequent infant complications.

Why it's important (chlamydia) If a mother has chlamydia, half of all babies who pass through her birth canal will get the infection, which could cause conjunctivitis or chronic pneumonia.

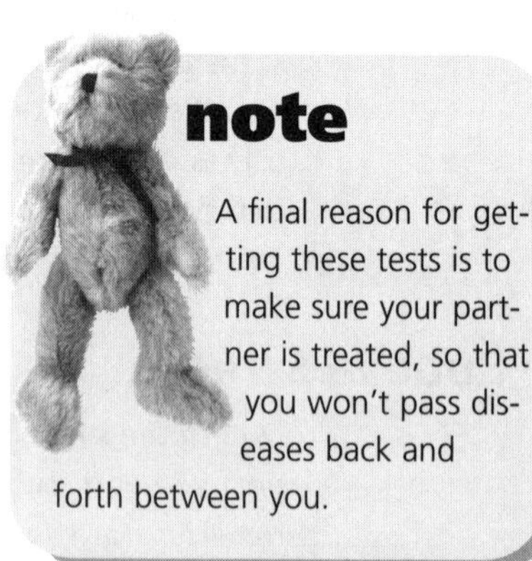

note

A final reason for getting these tests is to make sure your partner is treated, so that you won't pass diseases back and forth between you.

HIV Test for AIDS

It's been well established that there is a perinatal transmission risk of AIDS from mother to baby. In fact, the rate of passage to the baby is about 30%. Women who test positive for AIDS on their initial screening will be given a more specialized test called a *Western blot analysis*. If that tests positive, then a diagnosis of HIV infection is made and there are medications that can be given to reduce the risk of transmission to the baby. At this point, women are counseled as to how the infection can be spread and how transmission can be halted. In general, doctors frequently advise women who have AIDS not to get pregnant. Sometimes, they will even advise them to terminate their pregnancy because the mother's life could be at stake due to her immune suppressed state (she is overly susceptible to infections), and the baby's life can be compromised as well. There is a much higher risk for the mother to transmit the disease to the baby if her disease is severe or in an advanced stage of progression.

Interestingly, the HIV infection appears to have very little affect on the pregnancy, although the pregnancy itself can affect the degree of the HIV infection (making it worse) as it suppresses the immune system. There appears to be no advantage for having a C-section over a vaginal birth; however, many OBs are careful to avoid performing any procedures during labor that may increase the chances of fetal blood mixing with the mother's blood.

Why it's important: The baby may have the HIV infection, but not full-blown AIDS. AIDS is a deadly disease for the mother and baby.

note

HIV infection becomes AIDS as certain white blood cell counts fall, and the infected mother becomes more susceptible. When an individual is diagnosed with AIDS, the prognosis is poor with survival less than 2–3 years.

Approximately 10% of Americans who are infected with the HIV virus are women; and, unfortunately, this represents the group whose infection rate is rising most rapidly (over 50% of these women are of child-bearing age). Most women acquire the HIV virus through sexual contact and IV drug use. It's not surprising that over 80% of pediatric HIV virus is passed from mother to fetus.

More than 830,000 cases of AIDS have been reported in the United States since 1981. As many as 950,000 Americans may be infected with HIV, one-quarter of whom are unaware of their infection

GBS

Group B streptococcus is a bacterial strain present in approximately 20–25% of women. GBS poses no threat to the mother, but to a baby it can be lethal. The GBS test is designed to screen for those mothers who may be carriers for this bacteria. Most OBs recommend doing a culture from the vaginal and rectal area at about 36 weeks of pregnancy. If the test is positive, antibiotics are given at the time of labor to reduce any possible infection to the newborn. Antibiotics will also be given to women in preterm labor or if they have ruptured their bag of water for a prolonged period of time.

Why it's important: GBS infection is a common contributor to sepsis of the newborn, and it can carry a high mortality and morbidity rate for the baby, especially if the baby is born prematurely. However, sepsis of newborns occurs in less than 1% of all births, so it is considered rare.

Gestational Diabetes

Approximately 2–3% of women will develop gestational diabetes in their pregnancy (meaning that the pregnancy caused their diabetic condition). Generally, these are women who have no history or risk factor for diabetes. Because of this fact, a glucose screen is performed on most women in their third trimester between 26–28 weeks.

If you're having this test, you will drink a 50-gram oral glucose load (about a cup) and then have your blood sugar tested one hour later. There is no need to prepare for this test (such as fasting). If the test comes back abnormal, then you will be a candidate for a three-hour glucose tolerance test (GTT). Generally, this means you'll need to fast before the test is given, and some doctors will have you adhere to a special diet before the test is given. If the three-hour GTT is abnormal, then you will have a diagnosis of gestational diabetes, and it will be managed accordingly. Usually, the doctor will start with diet control, but you may need to be placed on medication or possibly insulin therapy. Often, gestational diabetes will disappear after the baby is born; however, sometimes it uncovers the potential for developing diabetes later in life. So, if you're diagnosed with this condition during pregnancy, it's a good idea to keep tabs on it with your doctor in the future.

Why it's important: Towards the beginning of the third trimester, the mother's body undergoes a good deal of stress and her ability to balance her sugars is tested to a greater extent. The maintenance of sugar balance affects her metabolism and her blood pressure, but it's a two-pronged effect, affecting both the mother and the fetus.

A mother with uncontrolled diabetes has the potential of causing a rapid growth rate in the fetus. This occurs because the elevated blood sugars in the mother are registered as elevated blood sugars in the baby. In a futile attempt to control the mother's blood sugar in the pancreas of the baby, the baby's pancreas increases insulin production. (Insulin is a growth hormone, and one of its primary effects is to control elevated blood sugar levels.) This fetal growth increases the likelihood that the baby won't fit through the mother's birth canal, due to its larger size. In addition, shortly after birth, the baby who has been programmed to crank out extra insulin is still producing extra insulin after the cord is cut, but it no longer needs it. So the baby could become hypoglycemic as its blood sugar plummets. This condition could lead to metabolic problems in the baby, affecting its future growth and development.

Optional Routine Tests

There are a couple of tests that are considered to be fairly routine, yet warranted if the mother's history indicates it. They are still considered to be routine tests.

Multiple Marker Screen

The multiple marker screen is a test offered to most pregnant women between 15–20 weeks. It is used to identify those fetuses with certain chromosomal abnormalities and also neural tube defects. The test is not inclusive of all chromosomal abnormalities, but it does look for the more common ones, such as Down syndrome. If the test is abnormal, then the patient may be offered a comprehensive ultrasound of the fetus, as well as the opportunity to have an amniocentesis.

Many times, this multiple marker screen test comes back abnormal because of a mistake in the dating of the pregnancy. The test is supposed to be performed between 15–20 weeks. If you are tested inadvertently at 14 weeks, the test may flag an abnormality that isn't really there. In this case, the doctors are trained to verify the dates as best they can before they proceed to an amniocentesis. Sometimes, they'll recalculate the dates to make sure they were accurate or look for minor errors. They'll probably do an ultrasound to measure the baby's gestational age. If they still believe the test result is abnormal, they may recommend other options.

note

In an amniocentesis, a needle is placed through the mother's abdomen and into the amniotic sac using an ultrasound to guide it. A small amount of amniotic fluid is retrieved and sent for analysis to verify the possibility of Down syndrome or one of the other common genetic abnormalities. The test can also look for neural tube defects, which includes spinal bifida or some other serious neurological abnormality. The test itself does carry some risk, including fetal injury or death, but this is very small, less than 1%. Still, the possibility should be discussed with your doctor.

Cystic Fibrosis Screening Test

This test involves a simple blood test for the mother and basically tests you to see whether or not you are a carrier of cystic fibrosis. If the test is positive, then the doctor will probably want your partner to come in for a test. The results of both parents' tests determine if the fetus is at risk for CF.

VALIDITY OF TESTS

Both of the above tests are optional, and the mother may determine whether or not she wants to take either or both tests. There are limitations to any test, so don't have unrealistic expectations. There is no perfect test, but in most cases, the available tests for these conditions are reasonably accurate. It's up to the woman and her partner what they do with the outcomes of these tests with input from their doctor.

"I am aware of cases where a patient's fetus has tested positive for an abnormality, and the baby didn't have it," says Dr. John. "Remember that the multiple marker screen is just that—a screening test, meaning that it is designed to pick up as many abnormalities as possible for the large number of pregnant patients in a given population. Because of this fact, there are inherent problems with accuracy. The test serves its purpose by screening a higher risk population and giving them the opportunity to undergo a more definitive and accurate test, if they so desire. Although the majority who receive the test are 35 years of age and older (because of increased likelihood of chromosomal abnormalities), the actual number of babies diagnosed with this condition is greater for women who are younger simply because there are more women in this age range having babies."

High Risk Tests

In addition to the routine history, the doctor will check for any unusual or serious medical conditions that the patient may have or that could be genetically related. For example, if you have a history of diabetes, sickle cell anemia, tuberculosis, blood clots, high blood pressure, previous abdominal or surgical history, or anything that might show up as a warning signal, your doctor will be paying closer attention to these areas.

Ultrasound

Ultrasound can be a routine test, but it can also be a high risk test when the doctor is evaluating a specific high-risk issue, such as pre-eclampsia, intrauterine growth restriction, placenta previa, and so forth. Sometimes, diabetic patients will have cardiac anomalies affecting their fetus, and this can also be monitored with ultrasound.

You'll find lots of controversy among doctors about the frequency of doing a routine pelvic or obstetrical ultrasound. Many women seem to take it for granted and would be happy to have one at every visit, but from a medical perspective, it's not necessary to get an ultrasound more than once or twice during the pregnancy (or even that often) without a medical indication.

The benefits of ultrasound include a more accurate dating of the pregnancy and a possible identification of any abnormalities sooner rather than later. For the most part in the U.S., routine regular ultrasounds have not been shown to improve the pregnancy's outcome or proven to be cost effective. Conditions where it might be medically indicated include when the fluid level is low or the baby is in a breech presentation; if the placenta is in an abnormal location; or if the doctor needs a special anatomic evaluation of the baby.

People often want to know the sex of their baby. If the doctor's schedule permits, she may accommodate the request for sex identification, but remember that it does take time and money for an ultrasound, so that's why it's not performed routinely for nonmedical reasons.

ULTRASOUND TO GO

Several years ago, ultrasound clinics were popping up in malls. The clinic would offer to make a videotape of the baby for you (for cash, of course). It was strictly done for fun and for the parents' personal video collection. However, some babies were born with anomalies that were not detected, and the mall clinics were sued. That was the end of the mall clinics.

Don't worry about the safety of ultrasounds. They've been around the U.S. for decades, and no adverse effects on babies have been detected thus far.

The downside to an ultrasound is that the ultrasound itself is only as good as the equipment and the sonographer or person who interprets it. Sometimes, there is an anatomic anomaly that is present, but in the early stages of pregnancy goes undetected. You simply can't see all the problems that may be there, so it's not a foolproof method. The ultrasound merely shows you an image; it doesn't reveal the microscopic changes in the structure of organs. Dr. John describes it as looking at a vast field, and looking for a hole out there that is covered with grass, so you can't see it, meaning that he is looking for specifics, while the parents are enjoying the view.

Other High Risk Tests

Whatever medical conditions or history a mother has will dictate specific tests to evaluate those concerns. Some conditions might necessitate testing for heart disease, severe diabetes, high blood pressure, neurological problems, renal disease, cervical and/or uterine abnormalities, thyroid dysfunction, asthma, lupus, breast cancer, cancers in general, and frequent miscarriages. These are just a few potential medical problems that may require further medical investigation, as these conditions have the potential for adversely affecting the mother's health, as well as the baby's. It's important that you be honest with your doctor and let him/her know all your past medical and surgical issues (and family histories) that you may have been exposed to. Your baby's life and your own could be at stake.

THE ABSOLUTE MINIMUM

When a doctor orders a test, it's not done superfluously—there is a reason behind it. Be sure that you are honest and forthright with your doctor or midwife when it comes to your medical history so that they can give you and your baby the best care possible.

- Most women will be given an array of medical tests in the beginning of their pregnancy so the doctor can be better informed about their medical condition.
- If your health care professional suspects a problem at any time, he or she will order more extensive testing to evaluate your condition and your baby's health.
- Don't be afraid to question the doctor's reasons for giving a test. It's your right to know what the doctor is looking for.
- Be up-front with your doctor about your medical history and anything that might affect it. Lives are at risk—yours and your baby's.

PART iii

Second Trimester

IN THIS CHAPTER

- Physical changes that you'll notice
- Psychological changes that you may experience
- Questions the doctor will ask you about your progress
- Wearing maternity clothes

10

SECOND TRIMESTER—MOTHER

The pregnancy is moving along and soon you'll be at the halfway point. By now, you've probably adjusted to the fact that you *are,* in fact, pregnant; it's not going away, and soon you'll have a new life in yours. The excitement is starting to build as your body changes and grows. The second trimester is a "lovely" (says who?) time in the pregnancy. You're not too large to enjoy doing many of the same activities you did while not being pregnant, yet you're big enough for everyone to remark on your condition and share the joy with you (translation: make fun of you).

Physical Changes

Of course, your most obvious physical change in the second trimester is that increased expansion of your uterus—meaning the baby is growing, and you're expanding in size to accommodate it. Up until now, you probably haven't had to put on maternity clothes, perhaps only loosening your belt a little. This is the time to break out the new clothes. As you gain weight during this trimester, it will all seem to go to your fast-disappearing, former waistline, now slightly resembling a beach ball.

THAT ITCHY BELLY AND STRETCH MARKS

Along with that expanding belly, comes stretching skin. It seems as if the more the skin stretches, the "itchier" it gets, almost as if the skin is popping from its seams. Scratching doesn't really do any good. The best remedy is to use creams to alleviate the dryness of the skin.

Stretch marks are a common occurrence during pregnancy. Be prepared for them. Stretch marks can vary in color, ranging from purple to pink initially, but eventually they become silver or white. They usually appear on the lower half of the abdomen, but also can occur on the breasts and thighs. At present there is no effective treatment to prevent stretch marks from occurring. In addition, it's very difficult to eliminate them once they have appeared. Surprisingly, stretch marks are not caused by weight gain, but are usually the result of the stretching of normal skin. There is very little you can do to prevent them, and there may be a genetic predisposition or component to whether or not you get them. Or you may not get stretch marks from the one pregnancy, but will get them on others.

Your blood volume will continue to expand. This is a continued effort to increase the amount of blood flow to the uterus and the developing baby. In addition, the increased blood volume will compensate you, the mother, for the blood loss you will experience after the baby is born.

Your blood pressure should go down slightly because the vascular system has less resistance to blood, and the blood vessels are relaxing to allow more blood to flow through. This is a good thing, as long as your blood pressure doesn't get too low. If it's too low, it can reduce the blood flow to the baby. Because of the vascular changes, it's a good bet that you may feel dizzy from time to time, especially as you sit or stand up from a lying down or prone position. This dizziness will pass as your body adjusts to the new change in position, and blood flow is restored to your brain.

Your respiratory rate is increasing slightly during this time. There can be a perception that you're not getting enough oxygen, but the truth is that you're taking more breaths, and you're actually getting as much air as your body requires. You may find it harder to breathe because there is more compression of the diaphragm as the uterus displaces other organs, such as the intestines, liver, etc. This is normal.

Ever notice that pregnant women walk slightly differently than other people—almost as if they're walking a tightrope at all times? In many ways, they are. Your balance will be altered as your abdomen starts to project outward. And your shoulders will lean backward to compensate for the change in your center of gravity. You may also have more back discomfort and pain during the second trimester. Part of the reason for the pain involves your change in posture, but it could also be from the hormonal changes affecting your ligaments. The hormone relaxin prepares the birth canal by loosening the ligaments so the baby can pass through it. Because of this loosening in the pelvic region, the back doesn't receive as much support as it used to—ergo, the pain. It's particularly vital to practice good lifting habits at this time, since you could easily injure or put out your back.

tip

Good lifting habits can prevent injury at all times. Try to lift with your legs instead of leaning over and putting all the pressure on your back muscles. By squatting and using the power in your legs, you are less likely to pull a muscle in your back. Of course, the best advice is to lift as little as possible during this phase of the pregnancy.

Remember that the better the shape you're in before the pregnancy, the less likely you'll be to have pain and discomfort during the pregnancy. It's well known that strong abdominal muscles can help support the back, and being flexible and not overweight will reduce unnecessary strain on the back muscles. Keep exercising and staying fit!

Often, women experience wrist or hand pain, which might be caused by carpal tunnel syndrome. Carpal tunnel can occur as the woman retains more fluid and the fluid may compress and entrap the nerves in the wrist. Doctors think this can be attributed to hormonal changes, but they're not entirely certain of all the reasons. About 10–15 percent of women who get this condition may require some surgical treatment. It is actually pretty rare, though. You may be able to handle (pun intended) the situation by using wrist supports and avoiding repetitive wrist motion, such as typing on a keyboard (as the author could tell you).

Urine production is way up during the second trimester, so you'll be making frequent trips to the bathroom (if you haven't found that out already). The uterus has a compression effect on the bladder, making it feel more full, even when it might not be full.

Sleeping will start to get more and more uncomfortable the further you get into the pregnancy. In the last trimester, doctors advise women not to sleep on their backs.

During the second trimester, you should start trying to sleep on your side. The reason for this is that the great vessels (the vena cava and aorta) that carry the blood back to the heart run along the spine. The uterus can compress these vessels, allowing blood to flow more slowly, which will make you feel nauseous, light-headed, and could reduce the flow of blood to the baby.

tip

If you find it hard to sleep on your side, invest in a full-length body pillow that you can hug to your front to help you sleep if necessary. Or you can prop it against your back. Do whichever works best for you and makes you feel better.

Psychological Changes

The psychological changes that occur during this three-month period will vary from one woman to the next. Doctors aren't clear exactly what causes these psychological shifts, but the blame still obviously remains those pesky hormonal rises that occur throughout the pregnancy (heck, throughout your life is more like it!).

At times, you may feel as if you're under a lot of negative stress that is tough to deal with, perhaps crying more frequently or experiencing mood swings. Some women have issues with their changing bodies, as they put on weight. Other common problems that might exacerbate your mood include the following:

- Fears about the upcoming pain in labor
- Worries about your ability to deliver a baby vaginally
- Fears that the pregnancy isn't normal or progressing properly
- Concerns about being a good mother
- And, of course, all the normal stressful things that occur in anyone's life, such as how will the baby affect my marriage, my life, can I afford it, and so on.

FROM THE DOCTOR'S PERSPECTIVE...

Life is especially tough, I think, for pregnant women who aren't married, since they don't usually have as much security or financial and emotional support. However, even the most emotionally secure patient is worried about something, which is all very normal. In fact, I would worry more about a patient if she didn't express any concerns about some of these issues.

As a physician, I watch my patients with a history of depression even more closely as they progress through the second and third trimester. I try to gauge their mental and emotional well-being because I know they'll experience stressors, and I worry about a relapse of depression. If I identify specific issues during the pregnancy, then I'll try to get the patient an appropriate referral or consider putting them on an anti-depressant medication.

What to Expect at Your Doctor's Visits

In the second trimester, the visits to the doctor become more regular, occurring every four weeks on average (assuming a normal pregnancy). The doctor will check your vital signs, heart rate, and blood pressure, do a urinalysis (checking for protein or glucose), and review your symptoms and ask you how you're doing. The doctor might ask you general screening questions, such as "Have you had any bleeding? Is the baby moving all right? Have you experienced any problems?" This is the time when the doctor will review any outstanding tests you might have taken and discuss their results with you.

LEG SWELLING

What pregnant woman has not experienced swelling in her legs? Probably, not many, would be our guess. Doctors understand that swelling of the legs and hands is a normal part of pregnancy; however, doctors are very interested in knowing if a woman is experiencing any unusual pain in one or both of her legs. If you are experiencing pain or redness or unequal swelling, this could be a cause for concern. Deep veined thrombosis (DVT) occurs when a clot forms in the blood vessels, and pregnant women are at increased risk for this. The danger is that if a clot were to break off, it could travel up toward the heart and lungs and cause a potential cardio-pulmonary incident that could be fatal. Fortunately, this condition is rare, and is more likely to occur in the postpartum phase of pregnancy, especially after a cesarean section. So notify your doctor immediately—day or night—if you're experiencing these symptoms of redness or swelling, or go to the hospital immediately.

Next, the doctor will check the fundal height of the uterus by taking a tape measure, placing one end over the pubic bone, and then measuring the distance from that point to the top of the uterus. The fundal height is measured in centimeters. After 20 weeks of pregnancy, the fundal height in centimeters should approximate the number of weeks of the pregnancy to indicate normal growth (that is, it would be 20 cm. at 20 weeks). The measurement is considered to be normal if it is plus or minus two to three centimeters (read more about this in Chapter 11).

SEATBELTS AND HAIR DYE?

Not only is it OK to wear a seatbelt, but it is recommended to wear one at all times. However, because you are pregnant, be careful where the seatbelt goes or is placed. The lapbelt should ride below your abdomen and not directly across the baby, but below and over your hip bones. The upper portion of the seatbelt should ride normally across your chest and between your breasts.

Very little is known about hair dye and perms. They are probably OK, but most doctors would suggest not to subject yourself to chemicals during your pregnancy. So avoid the hair dye and perms if possible. Also, your hair may be a different texture during pregnancy, so it may react to chemicals differently than it normally would.

Break Out the Maternity Clothes

If you haven't already started wearing maternity clothes, chances are good that this trimester will see you in them. Women react differently to wearing maternity clothes. Some people love them and take a lot of pleasure in their changing bodies. Other women simply hate them and put off the experience for as long as possible.

You might be able to make do in the second trimester with loose fitting clothes that are not specifically maternity clothes, such as pants or sweats with elastic waists or dresses that are loose fitting and don't have a waistline. But toward the end of the second trimester, you'll have to break down and purchase some maternity clothes. There are maternity shops in every major city, and most major stores (and even discount stores) will carry a maternity line. If you're a size 10 in regular clothes, start with a size 10 in maternity clothes and work your way down or up from there.

tip

Here are a few online sites that you might like to check out while shopping for maternity clothes: www.maternity-mall.com; www.naissancematernity.com (chic, hip L.A. stuff) www.duematernity.com; www.mimimaternity.com; and www.maternityclothingonline.com.

Maternity clothes used to be dreadful looking, but now that pregnancy is considered to be hip and not something to hide, manufacturers are making cute clothes that are fashionable. Don't go overboard on your wardrobe because you do only wear them for a limited amount of time. Buy a few staples that will get you through the next few months and make you feel good. Keep in mind that you can always sell the later at a garage sale, consignment shop, or on eBay, but you won't get nearly what you paid for them.

THE ABSOLUTE MINIMUM

The second trimester is aa—your changing body, your changing emotions, and that changing baby growing inside of you. It works best if you regard this interim, middle period in the pregnancy as a time for rest, relaxation, and preparation. Accept these changes and delight in them, and the time will pass quickly.

- During the second trimester, your body will feel as if it is growing exponentially and daily, as the weight gain increases, the baby gets bigger, and you notice different changes in the way you walk and feel.
- Be prepared for emotional ups and downs. It's normal to experience highs and lows during pregnancy. Stay calm, take deep breaths, and focus on the joy that is coming to you soon.
- Make sure that you keep tabs on your own body so that you can help the doctor better understand your condition at all times. Note if the baby is kicking and active. If you ever suspect that anything is wrong, alert your doctor immediately.
- Get some cute maternity clothes that are fun to wear and help you enjoy the experience.

In This Chapter

- How the baby is changing and growing inside of you
- How you'll notice that there is a baby inside of you
- How to spot signs of pre-term labor

11

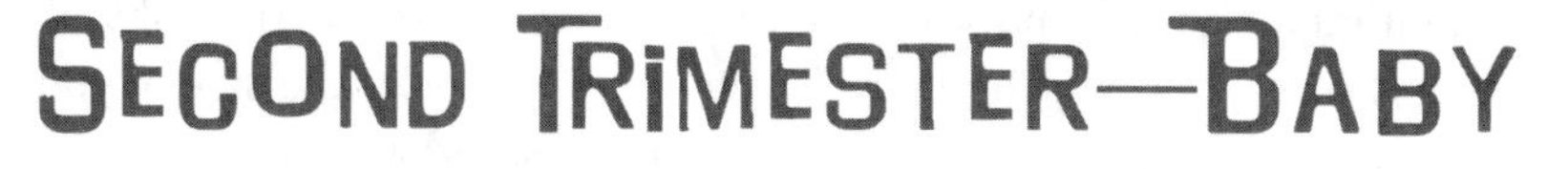

Second Trimester—Baby

By the second trimester (weeks 14 through 27), you'll know that there is a wonderful alien entity inside of you—that thing we call your *baby*. Lots and lots of things are happening to your baby during these three months. Mostly, it's growing, but you'll start to feel it kicking and moving during the fifth month. It's becoming a force inside of you with its own identity. And guess what—already you can't control this thing.

The Baby's Physical Changes

In the beginning of the second trimester (weeks 13 and 14), the baby is only about 4–4 1/2 inches long (the length of a writing pen minus an inch) and it weighs about 1 3/4–2 3/4 ounces, (put some weight on your postage meter to see exactly how small that is—about the weight of a couple of letters). The baby is covered by fine hair with blood vessels visible through the skin. The bones are hardening. Although it is extremely tiny, the fetus can smell, taste, swallow, and may suck its thumb.

Further along in the trimester, by week 19, the baby's length has increased to 5 1/4–7 1/4 inches long (slightly over half a ruler), and it weighs between 7–10 1/2 ounces (the weight of two bagels or a large orange). The fetus is starting to gain weight and put on fat, and it can now hear (so this is the time to play music for your baby). The fetus is also swallowing the amniotic fluid, which aids in its digestive system.

From 22–25 weeks the baby has grown from 8 3/4–10 3/4 inches and is between 1 1/2–3 pounds in weight. The baby looks more filled out (it's gaining fat), and it has eyebrows, eyelashes, and hair on its head. It appears to recognize the parents' voices and it might have a chance at survival if born this early. The baby also has sleep/wake cycles, which you will know from the kicking inside of you. Hopefully, the baby will be on a similar schedule to yours, rather than keeping you awake all night long partying inside of you.

By the end of this trimester, most of the baby's organ systems should be fully formed; however, there is still maturation occurring. This means that the heart and lungs are still growing and maturing to the point where the baby will eventually be able to function on his (or her) own. The lungs in particular aren't ready for the baby to be born, and the heart is still too small. The nervous system is showing the greatest changes at this point. The nervous system helps to regulate the baby's heart rate, as well as the movement of the baby's diaphragm muscles, which eventually will help the baby to breathe. The presence of breathing movement is a sign of maturation.

What You'll Notice First, and When

For most of us, having a baby is all about those landmark events that occur throughout the pregnancy. One of the most important and awe-inspiring occasions is when you first hear your baby's heartbeat. Although the baby's heart actually starts beating a few weeks after conception, you probably won't hear it until around the 12th week of pregnancy or later. In the old days, doctors used stethoscopes to hear the baby's heartbeat. Now, they do it with an electronic handheld device called a *fetal Dopplertone*, which has a speaker connected to it. It's positively amazing when the doctor or nurse rubs that transducer across your abdomen and all of a sudden you hear that tiny thumping vibration inside of you. Who would have guessed that a faint noise like that could give you so much joy and pride?

FROM THE DOCTOR'S PERSPECTIVE...
Sometimes, the mother will ask if I can tell if the baby will be a boy or a girl based on the heart rate (and old wives' tale). I usually say "no," because it's not a valid test. We're listening for 10–15 seconds, which gives us a snapshot of the baby's heart rate. I wish it were that simple to determine the baby's sex.

caution

Caffeine ingested by the mother can speed up a fetal heart rate. In fact, consuming more than 300 milligrams of caffeine daily has been linked to miscarriage. A Starbucks 16-ounce "grande" Breakfast Blend contains between 259 and 564 mg. of caffeine, so think twice before you drink your next cup, or try the smaller version. Because you metabolize caffeine even more slowly during the second and third trimester, it's best to avoid caffeine as much as possible during this time. Interestingly, in babies born to mothers who consume high quantities of caffeine, the baby is apt to experience withdrawal from caffeine when it is born.

The next banner moment occurs when you feel that first flutter of a kick, sometimes known as *quickening*. The first time it occurs, you will think you're imagining it or your stomach is having conniption fits with gas. It may also feel like a tickling sensation. But as the kicking gets more definitive and stronger, you'll recognize that amazing feeling of having a living human being inside of you (one who later seems to get a perverse pleasure out of kicking your guts out in the latter half of the pregnancy). The first signs of kicking generally occur between 18–20 weeks of pregnancy, depending on the fetus' size, activity level, and so on.

Your doctor may ask you to count the baby's kicks toward the end of the second trimester (see more information about this subject in Chapter 15). The idea behind the kick count is that the baby should have a given number of movements in a set period of time, simply due to the maturation of the baby's nervous system. Doctors feel that the kick count enables the mother to assess her baby's condition in-between office visits to the doctor.

KICK COUNT
One way to do a kick count is to choose a one-hour window, preferably when the baby is active. Then count how often the baby moves. Once you count 10 fetal kicks, look at your watch, and if it's been less than an hour, you're finished for the day. Your baby is well and active.

Some women may notice their baby hiccupping during the second trimester and into the third trimester. This can be quite disconcerting the first time it happens, albeit amusing.

During the second trimester, your doctor may decide that you should have an ultrasound exam to verify dates, growth, and the position of the baby. At this time, you can ask what the baby's sex is, if you're so inclined. An ultrasound may be performed as early as 13–14 weeks, but typically it is done between 18–20 weeks gestation to better evaluate the fetal anatomy.

During most of the second and part of the early third trimester, the doctor will also check how the baby is lying in the abdomen, whether it is breech (sideways) or head down. It's normal for a baby to be in the breech position for all of the second trimester and part of the third. Most babies will adopt a head-down position as they prepare for birth.

note

When the abdominal scan is done via ultrasound, the bad news is that you have to have a full bladder if the timing coincides with the early part of the pregnancy. Be prepared to do some squirming and hope that the people doing the test aren't delayed so that you have to wait.

Common Tests During the Second Trimester

Your doctor may order some blood tests during the second trimester. These tests may include a *multiple-marker screen* (MMS) that tests for the possibility of certain genetic disorders as well as spina bifida. This is generally considered an optional test because you, as a patient, may be faced with decisions that could affect the outcome of the pregnancy if the test results reveal that an abnormality truly exists (see Chapter 9). It's important to note that the MMS is just that—a screening test, which means that there is an associated false/positive rate. If the multiple-marker screen is abnormal, the doctor may recommend that you undergo an amniocentesis to verify the screening that indicates the baby may have a genetic disorder and/or spina bifida. The definitive test to verify or refute the screening results is an amniocentesis combined with a diagnostic ultrasound of the fetal anatomy.

Another test the doctor may order is a glucose tolerance test, which is a blood test that is performed at the end of the second trimester. This test checks for the presence of gestational diabetes (see Chapter 9) The doctor may also repeat your complete blood count test to see if you need additional iron; and, if you're RH negative, the doctor will check to see if you need a medication called *RhoGAM* (see Chapter 9).

Pre-Term Labor

Late in the second trimester is when signs or symptoms of pre-term labor are more likely to appear. Pre-term labor is the presence of *regular* uterine contractions combined with *cervical change*, which means that your cervix is starting to dilate as a result of contractions. This can be a very dangerous situation for the baby for obvious reasons. Keep in mind, though, that it's quite normal to have *irregular* contractions, also known as *Braxton Hicks contractions*. These contractions differ from regular contractions associated with pre-term labor in that they are irregular in frequency, duration, and strength.

Here are some signs of pre-term labor:

- Contractions (menstrual-like cramping)
- Gas-type pains
- Low pelvic pressure
- Low backache
- Blood from vagina
- Increased discharge from vagina

If you are having any of these symptoms and you're still not sure if you're in pre-term labor, then contact your doctor or health care professional immediately.

The Absolute Minimum

During your pregnancy, the second trimester can be one of your best times. You have tangible evidence that there is a baby inside of you, but you're not totally uncomfortable yet. Keep alert to signs and symptoms that the baby is growing and healthy inside of you. If you sense anything wrong, get help immediately.

- The baby is changing and growing rapidly during this trimester, so help the doctor monitor its progress by tracking kick counts.
- Eat right, get plenty of sleep, and continue drinking your water. What you do *does* affect your baby.
- Don't obsess about pre-term labor happening, but do be aware of the signs and symptoms.

In This Chapter

- What kind of physical limitations can you expect before delivery?
- Who will be present at the birth?
- How do you pick the right support person?
- What do I have to think about in advance of the birth?

12

Important Things to Decide Before the Baby Is Born

So, the baby is about three months off, and you're getting excited, but you've been dreading talking about the particulars with your significant other (who knows nothing), your mother (who knows everything), your extended family (who want to be included), and friends (who have their own agenda). Everyone has expectations centered around your baby. And being the dutiful daughter, daughter-in-law, wife, sister, friend, etc., you want to make everyone happy. Guess what—it ain't gonna happen. *You* are the important person here. Think about what *you* want to happen when you have your baby (and afterwards) and put your foot down. This is *your* baby, and it's your experience. The other people can just tow the line and fall in with your plans.

Physical Limitations

Make some advance preparations for the fact that you are going to have some physical limitations before and after the birth of your new baby.

Before the baby's birth, you will be extremely fatigued, due to hormonal changes and breaks in your sleep pattern, not to mention the fact that the size of your belly gets in the way of sleeping in a comfortable position. This would be a good time to get some extra help from family and friends if you want to clean the house or complete any projects.

> **caution**
>
> Don't forget to pay your bills during and after the pregnancy—with all the celebration and hullabaloo, it's an easy thing to blitz! Having a baby is tremendously exciting and takes priority over everything else, as you'll soon find out. Things seem to just go by the wayside. However, the bills keep coming, as does the mail. Arrange for someone else to handle the mail and the bills during this time because you will inevitably forget.

Avoid any activities that could jeopardize your health or the health of your baby, meaning that you don't want to fall, be injured, or traumatize your body in any fashion. Use common sense in your activities because you will be less able to get around. Let family members know that they may have to pick up some of the slack here, say helping with the gardening, housework, shopping, or other chores.

Be sure to line up help for yourself after the baby is born; for example, it's a great time for grandparents to be useful and welcome. Work out a schedule so that you're covered for at least the first few weeks after delivery—the longer, the better. Believe me, you won't want to tackle those weeks alone.

Here are some areas of your life that *will* change after the baby is born:

- You'll be very, very tired and need more sleep than usual. Plan on having someone in to help watch the baby so that you can get caught up on sleep. The baby could be up every couple of hours to eat, making a good night's sleep downright impossible.(Get used to it—it's going to last 20 years, give or take....)
- You won't be able to do your normal workload and activities for a couple of weeks. For example, you shouldn't carry or lift more than the baby's weight (or less). Light housework and exercise are OK, as long as you have the time and energy to do them. Slowly and gradually, you can return to a normal lifestyle after about a month to six weeks, but in the first few weeks, you simply shouldn't be doing much of anything. You'll still be bleeding from the birth, and your stitches need time to heal.

- Obviously, you can cook, but picking up the phone and ordering out might have even more appeal. If you're lucky, friends and relatives will keep you supplied with food. The only problem with cooking (other than cleanup) is that standing in one place for any length of time isn't always comfortable after having a baby. (Sometimes, you feel as if your guts are still spilling out.)
- If you had a vaginal delivery, you probably shouldn't drive for a few weeks or so. Plan on having someone else drive you around. It's too easy to tear your stitches if you get into a tight situation and need to brake suddenly. If you had a c-section, you won't be allowed to drive for a month to six weeks. You'll need help grocery shopping too, in this case.

tip

Exercise is good for you after you have a baby, although not strenuous exercise. Moving around and being somewhat active is important because not moving could cause blood clots.

Pushing a stroller and taking the baby for a walk accomplishes two things at once—the baby gets fresh air and you get exercise. Even c-section patients should walk. Dr. John's mantra: Drink water and walk; then walk and drink water.

Who's In, Who's Out

Here is the most important question, and also the most avoided question of any pregnancy: Who will accompany you into the labor and delivery room?

OK, there are really two questions here: Who do you want to be there during labor and who do you want to be there during the delivery? The labor and delivery rooms are often two separate places, although in many hospitals, the labor and delivery rooms are one and the same spot now.

Determine in advance which people are invited to experience which areas. For example, you might have frequent visitors coming and going during your labor, but you don't want them around during the delivery. Having people around to watch the labor is one thing; having them there to experience the birth might be too personal for you. Or you might not want anyone to see you in the throes of labor and delivery. That's alright, too.

If you want to confine your birth experience to you and your spouse (plus a few doctors and nurses), that's perfectly normal. As you near the actual delivery time, you just need to send all unnecessary people into the waiting room, so that you can experience the birth alone. Just let your nurse know your plans in advance, and she'll be the bad guy for you.

In general, you will have to follow the guidelines of the labor and delivery department of the hospital that you choose, so the number of people in attendance is really up to them (and their policies). Because of this, it's wise to visit the hospital early, look around, and check out how everything functions (see Chapter 3 for more details), so you don't have any surprises when you arrive. If you have questions, ask them in advance. Usually, labor and delivery rooms are among the friendliest places in the hospital.

In this hierarchy, the nurses manage everything in terms of your care (not the doctors). You will end up loving these nurses (male or female) who track their patients' needs at all times and establish who belongs in the L&D room and who doesn't. If you tell a nurse that you don't want an estranged boyfriend or ex-husband to be present, the nurse will keep them out.

Generally, when it comes time for delivery, the optimum number of extra people in the room is about two, in addition to the patient. The reason being that the space is small, and there has to be enough room for the doctors and nurses to perform their functions. Although medical personnel are sensitive to the patient's need for a support person, keep in mind that their first priority is to their two patients—mother and child. Everyone else is incidental.

FROM THE DOCTOR'S PERSPECTIVE...

In most births (vaginal deliveries), the extra person is the patient's significant other and maybe one other person, say a mother, sister, or close friend. However, I've been in deliveries where there were five extra people. I've also been in deliveries where there was just the patient. The important thing is to figure this out in advance, so there are no surprises or arguments at a time that should be happy. Then let the nurse know, and she'll handle the rest.

Choosing Your Support Person

If you are married, chances are your support person will be your husband. If you're not married, you might have other options. Pick your support person carefully. It should be someone who is calm because that person will have to keep you calm and peaceful when you're at your most agitated state. Your support person should also know you well and be the encouraging type, so that he or she can help you through potentially long hours of labor and delivery. Doctors and nurses rely on the support person to "translate" directions to the patient, who might not be at her best in terms of listening. Also, if the patient has any questions, often the support person will query the doctor or nurse for the patient, who, obviously, has more important things on her mind.

Don't be disappointed if your support person flakes out and doesn't really come through in the way you expected. This is probably a new experience for him or her as well. Even if your support person is just in the room to give you moral support, share the joy, or feed you ice chips—let's face it, passive support is better than nothing.

ONE PERSON'S SUPPORT IS ANOTHER PERSON'S ANNOYANCE

Your support person may be your best friend (or spouse) and the most wonderful person in the world, but during labor, he or she may bug you to death (for absolutely no reason). Keep in mind that you're not at your most charming when you're in labor. Little things can bug you a lot.

For example, Dr. John recalls when he was a resident hearing a woman in labor moaning, the nurse counting to 10, and then a slapping sound. Finally, he could stand the suspense no longer, so he went into the room and witnessed the woman in labor slapping her husband. That's right—slapping! The husband was looking like a nice, supportive husband who held his wife's head every time she had a contraction, but after she finished, she turned her head and slapped him across the face. Dr. John left the room and ran into the patient's mother-in-law. "I'm worried," she said. "Nothing to be worried about," said Dr. John. "The patient is doing fine." "I'm not worried about the patient," she said. "That's my son in there."

Meanwhile, the nurse called Dr. John back and asked when they were going to do a c-section. Dr. John was bemused and said, "What are you talking about, nurse? What would warrant a c-section?" "How about spousal abuse?" she replied with a smile.

If You Have a C-Section

If you have a cesarean section, then everything changes as far as who can watch the birth. Typically, only one additional person is allowed in the room for a c-section because you will be going into an operating room and a sterile environment. Additional hospital personnel will be necessary to take care of the mother and the baby because the risk is elevated. Also, more attention needs to be paid to the mother, and extra people would just get in the way.

In the case of a c-section, one extra person will be allowed into the room, but only in a mask, cap, and gown (sterile applies to everyone). He (or she) will be placed at your head, and there will be a curtain between your stomach area where the doctors are working and your line of sight. The extra person can look over the curtain and tell you what is going on, but you won't be able to see anything. Sometimes, the doctors are good about relaying information, but often they are busy handling the operation. The anesthesiologist will also be at your head during surgery, watching your vital signs.

Videotaping Your Future Star

Everyone has a different opinion about videotaping and photographing the birth, and hospitals have different policies, so it's wise to check out the policies first. Although you might think that you can get everything on camera, actually, that might not be the case. Hospitals will generally let you film before and after the delivery, but not necessarily during it. Blame the insurance companies and lawyers for this new rule, which is based on legal issues.

Pack Your Bags and Make Plans for a New Family Member

At the end of the second trimester, it's time to start thinking about packing your bag for the hospital. You don't need much, but you want to be ready, just in case. Pack this bag and put it in the trunk of your car, so you have it with you at all times.

Things to pack include the following:

- Toiletries
- Slippers
- An outfit to wear home, keeping in mind that it should be something loose and comfortable (you won't shed that weight as fast as you'd like)
- Nursing bras and underwear (preferably old, since you'll still be bleeding and might end up throwing them away)
- PJs or gown (again, you'll probably want to wear the hospital's gowns at least the first night, because you might end up staining anything you bring)
- Robe
- Favorite pillow
- CD player and music (if you want this in the labor room to soothe you)
- Baby clothes and blankets to carry the baby home
- Baby car seat
- Camera or video camera

Most importantly, make sure that you have a cell phone with you at all times, and that it is charged. You never know when you might have an emergency or your water might break. Be prepared. Cell phones are much more affordable today than they were before, so if you don't have one already, try to get one for a few months. There are some deals that are fairly cheap where you can just buy a designated number of minutes. Make sure your husband or support person also has a phone or a pager. And keep their number handy, either programmed into your phone or written down on paper. At the "pregnant" moment, you will probably be too excited to remember anyone's phone number.

Security

Hospital security is a big issue these days, so units will be locked and monitored at all times. You can expect secure doors, cameras, and special IDs (identification tags) on your baby that will trigger a monitoring system in the hospital to prevent infant abduction. When the mother delivers her baby, she will have an ID band placed around her wrist to match one that is also placed on the baby's wrist. Another ID will be given to the father so that he can be identified as related. Don't cut your IDs off until you go home.

tip

Don't take any valuables to the hospital, including rings, earrings, watches, money, wallets, etc. While a hospital is not the "hood," things do get stolen. Make sure that your husband or support person is responsible for any of your valuables, particularly when you change rooms. After you deliver the baby, you will be moved to a different room that will be yours for the rest of your stay.

Whenever you want to take the baby from the nursery, a nurse will check both your IDs before giving you the baby. These IDs will also be checked when you leave for home.

Choosing a Name

Now is a good time to start thinking about your baby's name, and there are numerous books out there to help you decide. (I'm sure every one of your relatives also has some ideas on this subject, and they won't hesitate to share if asked, or not asked.) Books can give you a description of the name you're interested in from a historical or religious viewpoint. If you don't know the sex of your baby in advance, then have a name picked out for a boy or a girl. It's not necessary to have the baby's name at the time of birth, but before you go home the hospital needs to know it so they can prepare and file the birth certificate.

FROM THE MOTHER'S PERSPECTIVE...

OK, I did not have a clue what to name my last baby (number 5—fresh out of names). Because she was born on July 4, 1986, she was given a Statue of Liberty nametag at the hospital, since the statue had just undergone renovations. The nurses tentatively called my new baby "Liberty." Hey, I even considered that name when after two weeks, the baby still did not have a name. By this time, the nurses were calling me frantically and were more than a tad peeved with me. The way I ended up picking my daughter's name was by going through our old family album and looking at last names for inspiration. I finally found a distant relation whose family lived in Vicksburg, and Vicksburg fell on July 4th to the Union army. It was enough of a connection for me.

Circumcision

If you have a boy baby, the doctors will ask you if you want to have him circumcised, which involves the removal of the foreskin on the boy's penis. This practice is fairly common in the U.S., but not as common in other countries. Sometimes, it is determined by your culture or heritage, although often the father seems to be the one to decide whether or not the baby will be circumcised.

There is a wealth of opinions, both pro and con about circumcision, and you would be wise to research the subject before proceeding. In the past, the procedure was performed to stave off infections, but many people feel that with today's health standards, it is no longer necessary. Most pediatricians will agree with whatever the parents want to do. If you want it done (or not), you should notify your family pediatrician, who will stop by the hospital to check the baby anyway. At this time, the procedure can be performed.

Parents will be counseled extensively about the risks of the procedure and must sign a consent form in order for the doctor to perform the procedure, which will take place in the nursery. Most of the time, the baby's foreskin will be anesthetized, so the baby doesn't feel any pain. The baby will be uncomfortable for a few moments when the anesthetic is given. Sometimes, the foreskin will come off immediately, but it may take a couple of days or a week or so to fall off.

IT'S YOUR DECISION

As a mother of three boys, I decided against circumcision, figuring that the boys weren't born that way and natural must be better. This was strictly my opinion and my husband's, but we did discuss it first with our pediatrician. Our doctor said that in today's society where hygiene is not an issue, circumcision is no longer necessary. Other pediatricians might feel differently. They might cite the fact that the boys will "look" different or might need to have the procedure done later in life when it would be more painful. My boys have never had any problems, and they are now grown. Moral of the story: Do your own research and make your own decision.

Breast Feeding

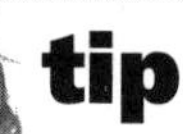

> **tip**
>
> The La Leche League International is a good resource for nursing mothers (`www.lalecheleague.org`), and will answer all your questions or point you in the right direction for answers.

By now, you should have an inkling of whether you will breast-feed or bottle-feed your baby. As soon as the baby is born, you will have an opportunity to feed the baby fairly soon. Doctors do stress that there is a wealth of information showing that breast-feeding has significant advantages for the baby over formula-feeding. Breast-fed babies have fewer problems with infections, bond better to the mother, and receive better nutrition, according to the research. Simply put, babies who breast-feed are healthier than babies who don't, which is why women are strongly encouraged to follow this practice. If for some reason you can't or don't want to breast-feed, let the nursing staff know so that they have a plan in place for bottle-feeding the baby.

If you're thinking about nursing your baby, most hospitals have lactation consultants who will help you get started and give you encouragement. Nursing a baby is not as instinctual as you might imagine, but both mother and baby can be taught. It can be painful in the beginning as you're getting started and used to it, but well worth it to persevere.

The Absolute Minimum

You're finished with the second trimester, and the baby's birth is getting closer. It's time to make some decisions about what will happen at your labor and delivery and afterwards when the baby is born.

- Get help. We can't say this often enough. Being pregnant and going through labor is not an excuse to wimp out, but it is pretty draining on your body. Call in the favors now.
- Pack your suitcase early. No sense in having someone else hunting through your things.
- Make sure your support person is indeed supportive and not a potential irritant.
- Get the "name-calling" between you and your significant other out of the way early and decide on a few names for your baby. This is one of those areas that you don't want to put off, as it can create some family dissension in the rank and file (and that's putting it mildly). Or, you could just wait to see what the baby looks like, but don't be surprised if that precious child is named Ernie (of Bert and Ernie fame) or Sponge Bob.

PART IV

Third Trimester

In This Chapter

- Still more of those physical changes occurring
- What can you do to alleviate the swelling and lack of sleep?
- What is pre-eclampsia?
- When and how labor is induced

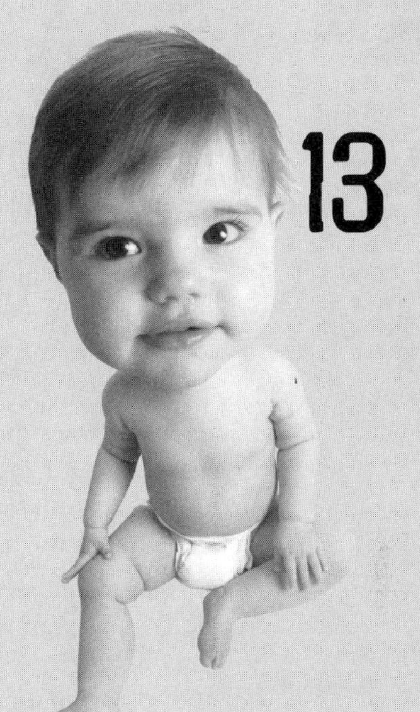

13

Third Trimester—Mother

OK, is there anything good to say about the third trimester? You don't like the way you look; you have no self-esteem; all of the excitement of the first trimester has transformed into desperation; even your maternity clothes are tight; and you have the attitude of a 6-year-old on vacation in the back seat of a car saying, "Are we there yet?" Despite all the negatives, one positive still looms large: Soon, you will have a baby!

You're in the Home Stretch

If pregnancy were a game, you'd be in the last third of a 40-week stretch, heading for the finish line. For the next 12–13 weeks your body will continue to grow and change. Besides the obvious fact that you're getting bigger in size and dimension, you're also encountering a few problems due to that size. First, your center of gravity has changed markedly, and it's more and more difficult to walk and maintain your balance.

Second, the swelling of your legs, feet, and hands becomes quite uncomfortable. Be sure to wear comfortable shoes, whether you're on your feet all day or not. In the evening, try to elevate your feet above the level of your heart. Doing this will help gravity keep the excess fluid from settling in your lower extremities. Take your rings off, if possible, since your hands will inevitably swell, and the rings might be unbearably tight.

Third, you simply aren't sleeping as well. The baby is awake and kicking while you're trying to sleep (it's more active in the first half of the third trimester), and you can't get comfortable to save your life. No sleeping position works very well for any extended period of time—that is, the time it takes to get a decent night's sleep.

SLEEPLESS IN WHEREVER

Sleep becomes a precious commodity when you're pregnant and sleep deprived. Dr. John wants to make it even more difficult for you. He says *never* to sleep on your stomach or your back during the latter third of your pregnancy because it compresses the baby's flow of oxygen. Not to get too specific or anything, but he wants you to sleep on your *left* side preferably. "When a pregnant woman lies on her left side, there is slightly more of a release of compression of the great vessels running along the spine and more of a profusion of blood to the uterus," he opines. OK, ladies, if you have to sleep on your *right* side (and I did), he says that is OK. Sheesh!

Other Physical Changes

In the third trimester, the doctor will be checking your blood pressure more often and continuing to monitor the growth of the baby via periodic fundal height checks.

DOCTOR'S VISITS INCREASE

From the beginning of the third trimester until weeks 34–35, you will be going to the doctor once every four weeks. From week 34–37, you'll start going every two weeks. After that, you'll visit the doctor once a week. The doctor will be checking your cervix for any complaints you might have regarding possible pre-term labor and giving you his best estimate of when you're going to deliver. (Never fear, they are usually wrong.)

The doctor will counsel you to do your kick counts on a regular basis. You'll notice more Braxton Hicks contractions, and it may become hard to differentiate between false labor and real labor. You may find yourself contacting your doctor more often about those "fake" contractions or going into the hospital to be checked, but likely you'll be sent home and told to wait.

You may notice an increased vaginal discharge, which is probably due to an increase in the amount of cervical mucous that is being produced. The consistency can range from thick to thin and almost watery. Sometimes, women get confused and think that their bag of water has broken when they see this mucous. It hasn't. Instead, what has probably happened is that the moisture you've noticed may actually be urine that has leaked out from your bladder due to direct pressure of the baby's head on the bladder.

The discharge could also be caused by an infection. The way to differentiate is that infections usually have a foul odor and may cause irritation in the vagina. If you're unsure which it is, mention it to your doctor. If you're diagnosed with an infection, antibiotics will be prescribed (they are considered safe at this stage of the pregnancy).

To make things even more confusing, there is another type of "discharge" that you might see. If you notice a large pinkish discharge, you may have dislodged the mucous plug. This is a good thing and means that labor is commencing. The mucous plug is the mucous that has been filling the cervical opening and is now dislodged due to the changes the cervix is undergoing as labor progresses. Usually, labor commences within days (if not sooner) of the mucous plug coming out.

Possible Pre-Eclampsia

Although swelling during pregnancy is normal, if you have swelling that is rapid in onset along with elevated blood pressure, then you might have a condition known as pre-eclampsia. Pre-eclampsia is a unique form of hypertension or high blood pressure associated with pregnancy. In the past, doctors primarily used swelling as a marker for the condition. Now, they focus on elevated blood pressures along with excess protein in the maternal urine. However, any excessive and abrupt swelling is not something to ignore and should be reported to your doctor immediately.

If your doctor thinks you might have pre-eclampsia, then the next step is to do serial blood pressure checks (meaning taking the blood pressure repeatedly over a period of time), do a thorough physical exam, and obtain some laboratory tests. If your condition is mild, the doctor may recommend bed rest. However, if you are close to term and have severe pre-eclampsia, the doctor will probably want to induce you. The only cure for pre-eclampsia known today is the delivery of the baby.

The exact cause of pre-eclampsia is unknown, although it can occur as early as 20 weeks into the pregnancy. For whatever reason, it's more common in first-time mothers and women at the extremes of reproductive age (teenagers and women in their late 30s or early 40s).

Inducing Labor

When you hear the term "inducing labor," it refers to the process by which labor is stimulated by way of medications either placed within the vagina or given intravenously. Inductions are commonly performed when the mother or fetus is at risk or there is a concern that prolonging the pregnancy could put either one of them at risk.

Although many women beg to be induced, inductions are not to be taken lightly, because the risks of complications are increased. The main complication, oddly enough, for an induction is a *failed* induction. If the induction doesn't work, then a c-section must be performed. A c-section exposes both the mother and baby to additional risks, compared to a vaginal delivery, so doctors are generally reluctant to perform an *elective* induction.

When you are undergoing an induction, be prepared for it to take a long time, by that I mean days. Remember that an induction is an attempt to simulate in a shorter period of time what normally would take days or weeks to occur. Your body simply may be unwilling or slow to kick in.

Using Medicine to Induce Labor

If the cervix is closed when an induction is initiated, the doctor will likely use prostaglandin-based medications placed in the vagina near the cervix. As the medications are absorbed, they have the net effect of "ripening" the cervix, or softening and slowly dilating the cervix. Once this has occurred sufficiently, pitocin is administered through an IV, which has the end effect of stimulating regular, forceful contractions. If your cervix is already dilated, the doctor may proceed to the pitocin stage without the vaginal medications.

"Natural" Methods of Stimulating Labor

Don't be shocked if your doctor "prescribes" intercourse with your husband. It's the oldest and most natural way of stimulating labor. However, it's not appropriate for all patients, so discuss it with your doctor first (as if any of us would—it's too embarrassing).

Sometimes, as you approach your due date or are past it, your doctor might perform a "stripping of the membranes" in order to stimulate labor. Your doctor should discuss this with you in advance of the procedure, which is performed while he administers a cervical exam. If the cervix permits (in other words, if it is dilated minimally), the doctor will insert two fingers, the index and middle, into the cervix and gently separate the bag of water surrounding the baby from the cervix. The intent is *not* to break the bag of water, but simply to loosen the attachments. This loosening has the effect of releasing various hormones, including prostaglandins, which have been known to stimulate labor.

FROM THE PATIENT'S PERSPECTIVE...

I had my membranes stripped several times, and after the first time was successful (i.e., the baby finally came), I begged the doctor to do it on subsequent pregnancies.

Actually, you can't even tell when the doctor is performing the procedure. Once I asked my doctor when she was going to get on with it, and she smiled and said the stripping was already done. However, be prepared for some serious cramping and contractions afterwards, almost like having your menstrual period. It's wise to remember, at that time, that you asked for it!

Another natural induction method can be as simple as breaking the bag of water if you are sufficiently dilated. The doctor does this at the same time that he examines your cervix—placing his fingers inside the vagina, up against the bag of water. Once there, he will check to verify that there is no umbilical cord present that could get injured, and he will make sure the baby's head is well applied to the cervix, which prevents the umbilical cord from slipping past the baby's head into the vagina once the water is broken (potentially dangerous). When that happens, it's known as a prolapsed cord.

FROM THE DOCTOR'S PERSPECTIVE...

Occasionally, a prolapsed cord will be diagnosed at labor and delivery after the baby's heart rate has taken a turn for the worst, as seen on the fetal monitor. The doctor will then proceed to check the cervix, evaluating whether or not the baby is going to deliver soon. And lo and behold, the doctor will feel a pulsating umbilical cord ahead of the vagina with the baby's head compressing the cord. This is an example of an obstetrical emergency. Traditional teaching for OBs is that when this occurs, you leave your hand inside the vagina, thus elevating the baby's head off the umbilical cord to relieve the compression effect, and you call for help—*FAST*.

The patient is then wheeled back to the operating room with the doctor's hand still inside the vagina while additional OBs perform an emergency c-section. They drape the patient with the doctor's hand inside of her, with the doctor usually underneath the drape. His hand is cramping, his fingers are sore, but he can't move his hand. If he doesn't continue to elevate the head off the cord, then the baby could suffer since the blood flow would potentially be compromised.

Dr. John has actually been stuck in this position. He was an intern in San Diego when it happened, and he had to lie underneath the drapes between the patient's legs until the chief resident could rescue the baby. It was only about 20 minutes, but it felt like an eternity.

If and only if all these conditions are met, the doctor will insert a small plastic device with a point at the end that will effectively break the bag of water. A gush of fluid typically follows, which is warm and normally clear. Occasionally, the fluid may appear like pea soup—green and thick. If this happens, it usually means that the baby has had a bowel movement in utero, which has mixed with the amniotic fluid. Frequently, doctors associate this condition with stress affecting the baby. Additionally, this condition can occur when the baby is past its due date.

TURNING THE OTHER CHEEK, LITERALLY

You know, there are tons and tons of funny stories that doctors and nurses tell about their patients in labor and delivery. So we thought we'd share one about a doctor. This happened one time when John was on call in Florida. He still chuckles when he recalls it.

Residents get very little sleep, so when they sleep they sleep soundly. One evening around 2:00 a.m., one resident was sound asleep after having just crashed an hour earlier, when he was awakened and told a woman was delivering right at that moment. He threw off the covers, pulled on his scrub pants, ran to the delivery room, and slipped on his sterile gloves and gown. As he was delivering the baby, the drawstring on his pants gave way, and the pants started to slide slowly down his rear end and around his knees. The poor, young resident, who wasn't wearing boxers or briefs (who knew?), was mortified, but didn't want to break the sterile conditions by pulling up his pants. Fortunately, he was covered in the front by his gown, but he ended up mooning the rest of the staff until the baby was delivered.

Needless to say, the nurses, normally quite excited by a delivery, were even more so this time. The resident was the talk of L & D for quite some time after that day.

THE ABSOLUTE MINIMUM

The absolute truth is that the third trimester doesn't *last* forever (although it feels as if it does), you will live through it (although you won't believe it), and you will end up having a baby (the proof is in the pudding). But getting through the third trimester is a drag, and there is no easy way around it.

- Do your part for the baby's health by observing and recording the kick counts.
- Keep drinking that water and elevate those feet anytime you can. Don't forget to get some exercise—at least walking, so that you're in shape for the delivery
- Be aware of your contractions, so that you can tell the difference between Braxton Hicks contractions (which feel real) and real ones (which feel really, really real).
- If you have an inordinate amount of swelling, let your doctor know immediately. Don't take any risks with your health or your baby's.
- If you can get your doctor to induce you the natural way, go for it. You might as well get this thing over with. The caveat being—your doctor knows best, so if he refuses, know that he has you and your baby's interests at heart.

IN THIS CHAPTER

- Physical changes that occur in the baby
- The importance of amniotic fluid
- Checking the placenta if you go past your due date
- The different levels of nursery care
- When something goes wrong with the baby

14

THIRD TRIMESTER—BABY

The third trimester is that magical period of time when you know for sure that you're going to have a baby soon. The flip side is that it's that scary period of time when you know that you're going to have a baby soon. As you prepare mentally, your baby is experiencing increased growth inside of you and also "preparing" to be born.

The Baby's Physical Changes

A great deal of growth occurs in the last trimester, although you will notice less during the last month when the growth rate slows down as the mother approaches term. Between 29–33 weeks, the baby will grow to be about 11–16 inches long (the size of a basketball, which is what it feels like inside of you), and weigh anywhere from 3–5 pounds. The next four weeks the baby will experience even more growth from 20 inches to 22 inches long and weighing anywhere from 6–7 1/2 pounds or more.

How the Baby Changes

The third trimester supports continued growth of the fetus, maturation of the organ systems, a change in the amniotic fluid volume, and a change in the baby's position.

The fetus will be adding fat and looking more babylike. All of the organ systems are fully formed. There is a gradual increase in the baby's ability to breathe on its own as the lungs and nervous system continue to develop. Actually, the lungs are not fully developed until 37–39 weeks. Most of the time, nurseries have very high success rates at taking care of babies born prematurely if they are born after 34 weeks gestation, the main problem being the undeveloped lung system of the fetus.

The baby's eyes are open in utero, and it's moving around and visibly swallowing. The baby is "breathing" in the sense that its lungs are expanding and the diaphragm is moving up and down (one of the neurological maturation indexes for development). Actually, the baby is exercising its lungs in anticipation of when it will breathe air. Up to this point, the baby has relied on oxygen in the umbilical cord to meet its needs.

The baby will swallow amniotic fluid, which is processed through its digestive system and comes out as fetal urine. That fetal urine is a major component of the amniotic fluid that surrounds and cushions the baby. The fluid will decrease in volume as the baby approaches birth.

The fetus that was formerly in a breech position usually will convert to a head-down position as the mother approaches term. Because babies need this time to get to the correct position, it's common for pre-term babies to have a higher risk of being in the breech position due to their gestational age. For this reason, doctors check the baby's position carefully when a mother is in pre-term labor.

Kick Counts Continue to Be Critical

The fetal movements that the mother has been experiencing in the second trimester will continue, but it's normal for the baby to move a little bit less as you approach term due to a couple of factors.

- There is less room inside of you, so there is less free space for the baby to move around.
- The amniotic fluid has decreased.

Although the baby's movements may be less frequent, it should still continue to move, and you should continue to monitor the kick counts present (see Chapter 15 for how to monitor your baby's kicks). If you fail to have the proper number of kick counts, call your doctor immediately.

Monitoring the Amniotic Fluid

The amniotic fluid is essential for the baby's health and well-being. If the bag of water were to break prematurely, this can precipitate pre-term labor, which can be associated with complications for the baby. Any time a woman thinks she has broken her bag of water, she should report this as soon as possible to a doctor. Not surprisingly, when the bag of water has broken, the amount of amniotic fluid surrounding the baby is decreased. When the amniotic fluid level is low, the baby has a higher chance of lying on its own umbilical cord, which is its lifeline.

DETERMINING IF YOUR WATER HAS BROKEN

When your water breaks, it may come in a gush (in which case it's evident that it has occurred) or a continual leak (in which case it's less evident). Typically, water will suddenly gush everywhere, and there is nothing you can do to stop it. You may notice an increase in the amount of pressure in your pelvis and an increase in uterine contactions.

When you go to the doctor to have this evaluated, the doctor will test the fluid present in the vagina for the presence of amniotic fluid. He may also do an ultrasound to check the volume of amniotic fluid surrounding the baby. If your bag of water has been broken for a prolonged period of time, you and the baby may develop an infection of the placenta and uterus, characterized by fever, uterine cramping, abdominal pain, and possibly a foul discharge. So this is another reason to go to the hospital when you think your bag of water is broken.

Testing the Placenta

As the placenta becomes more mature, it begins to calcify and may no longer function as well, which typically occurs around the patient's due date. When this occurs, the placenta becomes less efficient at transporting vital nutrients across its membrane to the baby, and oxygen transport may be affected as well. Women who go past their due date might be asked to begin antepartum testing, which checks to see if the placenta is working well enough for the pregnancy to continue. Although there are different kinds of tests, the nonstress test is the most common.

With the nonstress test, a belt is placed around the mother's abdomen and the fetal heart rate is measured for 20–40 minutes. The doctor will then interpret whether or not the baby is doing well (if adequate oxygenation is present). In addition, the doctor may also request an ultrasound to measure the volume of amniotic fluid that is present. By combining a nonstress test with an ultrasound measurement of amniotic fluid volume, both a short-term and long-term assessment of the baby is obtained. Assuming that these tests are normal, reassurance that the baby will be OK generally lasts from three to eight days.

DATING AND ESTIMATING GESTATIONAL AGE

The estimated date of confinement (or EDC) is just that—it's an estimate. When caculating one's due date, it begins from the first day of the last menstrual period and lasts 40 weeks. The overwhelming majority of babies are born either prior to or shortly after the EDC. The due date should be looked at more as a range between 37–41 weeks, which is considered normal.

If a baby is born either prematurely or past its due date, then the pediatrician will do an examination of the baby to estimate the baby's true gestational age. He does this by employing one of two methods. The Dubowitz exam utilizes a standardized scale to measure the gestational age by a neurological exam. They also may estimate the gestational age by using a Ballard scale. The Ballard scale evaluates neuromuscular maturity and physical maturity.

The Different Levels of Hospital Care for Infants

The neonatal care found in a hospital is referenced by certain levels, the lowest being Level I and the highest Level IV. For example, Level I is known as *basic care*. Most nurseries are considered to be Level I. Their care of newborns includes feeding, diapering, bathing, watching for problems, and assisting families in their preparation for going home.

Level II is also referred to *as specialty care nurseries* or *transitional care*. Essentially, this level provides additional care for babies who need more assistance than a Level I nursery can provide. For example, if the baby needs additional oxygen support, IV medications, or is born prematurely, then the baby might be sent to a Level II nursery.

The babies in Level III nurseries (also known as *subspecialty care or NICU—Neonatal Intensive Care Unit*) may require monitoring for sleep apnea (baby forgets to breathe), IVs or special medications, incubators to maintain body temperature, and feeding assistance (for example, tube feedings or other help). Most babies who weigh less than 5 pounds 8 ounces or are premature will usually go to a Level II or a Level III nursery for observation or treatment. NICUs also provide assistance with ventilator and respiratory needs for babies having problems breathing on their own. IV lines and special equipment monitor the baby's blood pressure and heart function. These facilities also handle the monitoring of a baby's condition if the baby is considered to be unstable or in danger of his health changing suddenly. In addition, NICUs give follow-up care after surgery.

LEVEL III NEONATAL UNITS

When babies are born with severe problems or complications, they are generally sent to a level III neonatal unit or nursery. In the U.S., level III nurseries have a very high success rate at taking care of babies born prematurely compared to community-based hospitals where there are fewer resources available. Level III nurseries typically handle intensive care infants who require round-the-clock attention and special equipment, particularly for respiratory needs. These special units are more commonly located in urban centers where there is a greater volume of babies born who might have complications.

If a woman finds herself in the unfortunate situation of having a prenatal complication during pregnancy and she is stable, she is likely to be transported from a smaller hospital to one with level III care. That way the baby can instantly receive the care it needs when it is born. In contrast, if the woman were to deliver a pre-term baby at a smaller hospital, then the baby might need to be transported to another facility with high-tech capabilities. Sometimes, the baby will be transported by helicopter or ambulance, depending on the severity of the case. Generally, though, doctors would prefer to transport the mother while the baby is still inside of her because it's healthier for the baby.

Note that these resources are only needed in extreme circumstances. Generally, most hospitals have level I and II neonatal care that is sufficient for most births.

The highest level of NICU (neonatal intensive care unit) is a level IV. These nurseries are usually found in children's hospitals, and they provide the highest level of care possible, which includes transplants, heart bypass, and ECMO (Extra Corporeal Membrane Oxygenation, which means oxygenation outside the body and can be used to support the heart or lung function in very sick babies).

THE NICU MEDICAL TEAM

A neonatologist is a doctor specializing in newborn intensive care who heads up the medical team taking care of your baby. Your baby may also be under the care of various specialists, including a neurologist, a cardiologist, a surgeon, etc.

Other people who might care for your baby include a primary nurse, a clinical nurse specialist, a respiratory therapist, a nutritionist, a physical therapist, an occupational therapist, a pharmacist, lab technicians, a chaplain, and a social worker.

Fetal Demise

No matter how hard a medical team works during labor and delivery to ensure a successful outcome, sometimes the baby is born dead or dies shortly after birth. The cause of fetal demise or death is usually unknown; however, sometimes it can be associated with umbilical cord or placental accidents, where the blood supply is interrupted to the baby. Other conditions that could affect the baby's life and result in death are infections or a genetic abnormality. Often, the diagnosis of why the baby died can be made after the baby is delivered with the use of various tests obtained from the baby or from the amniotic fluid. Unfortunately, the answer of why the baby's death happened is usually unknown.

The best course of action at this time is prevention. If you notice a decrease in the baby's movement or your kick counts are not present or being satisfied, then report these concerns immediately to your doctor. Having said that, Dr. John warns, "I always advise my patients that even if they get their kick counts, but the mother perceives that something isn't quite right, then that's good enough for me. Let me know immediately. I'd rather be safe with my patients than sorry, and I trust a mother's judgment."

FROM THE DOCTOR'S PERSPECTIVE...

Unfortunately, obstetrics is not always filled with good stories. OBs, myself included, have been in the awful position of having to tell a mother that her baby is no longer alive. While this is a rare occurrence, each time it happens, it is devastating news to both the patient and their family, as well as the doctors and nurses caring for her. In all of the cases that I have experienced, the mother usually reports that she noticed a decrease in the amount of fetal movement beginning several days prior to letting her doctor know. Most mothers also say that "The baby didn't move as much the last few days, but I thought everything was all right. I'm worried because the baby hasn't moved since yesterday." Don't wait this long because it could be deadly. Report any loss of movement to your doctor immediately.

THE ABSOLUTE MINIMUM

Stay alert to any changes in your body during this trimester. Be aware that pre-term labor is possible *and* dangerous if it happens too early. Monitor your baby's health inside of you, by being aware of the baby and your body.

- While the baby is growing and you can see the obvious outward physical changes, there are a lot of changes occurring internally. Stick to your healthful regimen so that the baby gets all its nutrients.
- Although rare, babies can die at this stage for no apparent reason. The best "cure" is prevention. Stay attuned to the baby inside of you and notice any changes in movement, particularly if it is decreased. Report them to your doctor immediately or get to a hospital.
- Rely on your own judgment to determine the condition of your baby, rather than friends' opinions. If you have a question about your medical condition, never hesitate to call your doctor first.

IN THIS CHAPTER

- How to differentiate between fake contraction and real ones
- What other symptoms indicate you are about to give birth?
- What is fetal kick count?
- Questions you'll be asked by the medical staff and why
- What happens if you're not in labor
- How to pack for the hospital

15

WHEN TO GO TO THE HOSPITAL

The obvious answer to the question "When do I go to the hospital?" is "When it hurts." However, this may not be as easy an answer as it first appears to be. As a new mother, you may not know when you're in real labor as opposed to fake labor. And it could hurt in either case.

Fake Contractions (Braxton Hicks)

Most women will experience "fake" contractions sometime in their pregnancy—not all women, but most. Fake contractions, more commonly known as *Braxton Hicks* contractions, are real, honest-to-goodness contractions of the uterus. They look real on a uterine contraction monitor. They feel real. But they're not *called* real. The difference being that they are irregular contractions, and they don't cause your body to go into labor or your cervix to dilate. True labor is contractions with cervical changes.

Usually, you'll start feeling Braxton Hicks contractions sometime in the second trimester, getting more pronounced the farther along you go in pregnancy. They can feel like a tightening of the stomach, as your abdomen (or rather the uterus) gets hard for no reason. You'll know it when you feel it. If you touch the stomach with your hand while one of these contractions is occurring, it feels like a tight drumhead. There is no way to control the contraction. It will usually pass in a few seconds. In the meantime, just breathe your way through it. Or try changing your activity or drinking some water to alleviate the tightness.

Braxton Hicks contractions can be triggered by something as simple as the baby moving or someone merely touching your stomach. Although they are often called *practice contractions*, they don't actually play a part in dilating or effacing the cervix, like real contractions do.

Typically, Braxton Hicks contractions are not especially painful, but more uncomfortable than anything. These contractions may vary from a few seconds to half a minute, and you can't predict when they will occur. You may have a run of three or four contractions an hour, and then they will just stop for no reason. They might not come back for weeks, or they could come back an hour later. Go figure.

FROM THE DOCTOR'S PERSPECTIVE...

Since people have different pain thresholds, some women do describe Braxton Hicks as being very painful. When I ask a first-time mother to rate the pain, she may say it's a "10." Because she hasn't experienced labor yet, that pain is indeed a 10 to her. Usually, when that same woman goes into labor, she'll say that it hurts worse than Braxton Hicks, ergo the pain is now off the charts. Be aware that other factors may contribute to the intensity of your perception of "painful" contractions, anxiety being one of those conditions. Try to rest and minimize the stress in your life.

Having said that, the caveat is to always consult your care provider if you're in extreme pain. The pain could be coming from another source, like the bladder, yet feel as if it's in the same location as the uterus. Or it could be coming from a pulled muscle or a gastrointestinal problem and needs to be investigated further. Don't live with unnecessary pain. Make sure that nothing else is wrong.

Real Contractions

In comparison to Braxton Hicks contractions, real contractions are regular in duration and regular in their interval spacing. As labor progresses, they get more intense and last longer. For example, they may start off lasting a few seconds and occurring 10 minutes apart, but every hour they get closer and closer together and last longer. On average, a real contraction lasts from 30 seconds to one minute each. Typically, you'll start off with four to six contractions in one hour. When you have four to six contractions for two hours in a row, it's time to panic and call the doctor. Chances are good that you're in labor!

Real contractions can be anything from a dull ache and a tightening of the uterus (à la Braxton Hicks) to all-out, excruciating, gut-wrenching, eye-popping pain. Believe me when I say that you'll know it's the real thing when you experience them.

When contractions start, you should time them with a stopwatch to see how long they last. Then time them again to see how far apart they are. The doctors, nurses, and hospital personnel will all ask you these questions. "How far apart are they? How long do they last?" Get your partner to keep a chart of the contractions. This will often help the doctor determine over the phone if you need to get to a hospital, and if you're close to delivery. Nobody wants you to have that baby in the car, least of all your partner.

Be prepared for the contractions to change quickly, meaning that they can go from easy and manageable pain to over-the-top and unremitting, wrenching pain in what seems like an instant. When this happens, it means that the baby is progressing down the birth canal.

WHEN MINUTES COUNT

With my second pregnancy, I decided that I was an expert. After all, my first baby had been born one year earlier so I felt as if I knew everything there was to know. Babies took time to be delivered, didn't they? When the contractions started, I calmly informed my husband that I was going to "get clean" for the baby (and the doctor), so I stepped into the shower, figuring I had hours to go before delivery. Within minutes, I was doubled over in pain. My husband screamed at me to get out of the shower, which I did post haste. We barely made it to the hospital before I delivered a baby boy (thankfully in a room). My husband missed the delivery—both he and the doctor were still in the process of walking in from the parking lot. Time from actual first contraction to delivery—47 minutes. Moral of the story: Make sure it's a quickie—shower, that is.

Other Symptoms of Impending Birth

Besides the obvious contractions, you may feel increasing pain or pressure on the lower back, as well as the abdomen, as the baby moves down into the birth canal and into position. You might also think you need to have a bowel movement when you don't really have to go to the bathroom, or you could feel like pushing (don't go with that feeling quite yet).

Emotionally and mentally, you may feel distracted or distraught and unable to focus. You might be supersensitive emotionally and feel like crying a lot. You could also experience extreme fatigue, or the opposite, tons of energy. Swings of emotions can be attributed to many reasons. They could be caused by a lack of sleep, your diet not being as good as it is normally, stress, or even the fear of the unknown (for example, a first-time mother might be worried about the upcoming pain of labor and delivery).

You could act differently for any number of reasons or just from the daily problems of living. Most of the time, these feelings are quite normal. Usually, what helps is to have a good conversation with someone whom you trust and love who cares about you. Talk to that person and ask him/her to listen. A sympathetic ear goes a long way.

With questions specific to pain, you should talk to your physician or midwife so that your fears can be allayed. In modern obstetrics, the overwhelming majority of women will receive some form of anesthesia, so the pain of labor and delivery is much less intensified and not a cause for concern.

FROM A MOTHER WHO HAS BEEN THERE...

The worst time for me was always right before the baby came. I got tense, irritable, and asked my doctor nonstop when the baby was coming. I worried about everything from whether the house was clean to how I'd handle my in-laws to what to pack for the hospital. I worried about my body—would I be "fat" forever, would I still be attractive and normal after the baby was born, would my breasts sag, would I have stretch marks, etc. What I didn't do was stop to take a breath and calm down. I'd strongly advise that. Just an FYI—once the baby is born, all those pressures and tension are gone magically and instantly. It's a wonderful thing.

Fetal Kick Count

Important, important, important—this can't be stressed enough! Always be aware of that baby inside of you and its movements. One way to keep track of the baby is through the *fetal kick count.* The fetal kick count is determined by counting how many times the baby kicks in two hours out of the whole day. Here's how it works. Pick a one-hour window, preferably when the baby is active and count how often the baby moves. Once you count 10 fetal kicks, look at your watch, and if it's been less than an hour, you're done for the day.

If you don't get 10 kicks in one hour, you can extend the time period to two hours. If you still don't get 10 kicks, it's probably a good idea to go into your doctor for an evaluation.

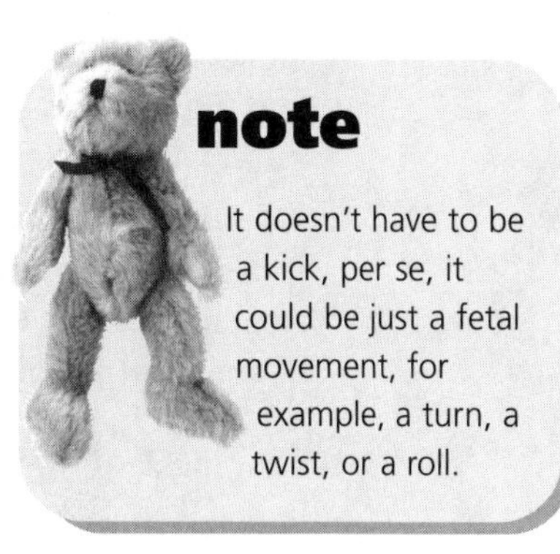

note

It doesn't have to be a kick, per se, it could be just a fetal movement, for example, a turn, a twist, or a roll.

The fetal kick count is simply a way for you to do a daily check of your baby's well-being in between doctor's visits. Studies have shown that when mothers don't get their kick counts tallied, it could make a difference in the outcome of the baby's welfare.

As you get farther into the third trimester, you may feel as if the baby is taking longer to get its kick counts, but you should still be able to get them. At this point, the baby is moving and active, but not as much.

FROM THE DOCTOR'S PERSPECTIVE...

Having said this, I always advise my patients that even if they get their kick counts, but perceive that something is wrong, they should come see me. I trust my patients' instincts and will have them come in for an evaluation anyway. Hey, it may look as if everything is going well with the pregnancy on paper, but if the mother feels something is wrong, it's worth respecting. A mother's intuition is usually right.

Get Thee to a Hospital

At any time close to your delivery date, if you think you're in labor, call your doctor or midwife. They will give you explicit instructions on what to do. If they tell you to go to the hospital, here is what will happen.

The hospital will be expecting you because the doctor will call ahead to alert them that you are en route. Go straight to the OB/GYN labor and delivery area where you will be evaluated. A labor and delivery nurse will check you first. She'll (or in some cases he'll) check your vital signs (blood pressure, temperature, pulse, and respiratory rate), and she will put external monitors on your abdomen. The monitors consist of a fetal heart monitor (a Doppler monitor), which measures the baby's heart rate, and a uterine contraction monitor (tocometer), which measures the duration and frequency of your contractions.

After about 15–20 minutes, the medical staff will be able to interpret the tracings from the monitor to determine if you are having real contractions, how many, and how closely spaced apartthey are. If you're watching the monitor, you can see the needle trace your contraction pattern.

With the record that the fetal heart monitor provides, the caregivers can determine what the baby's condition is and his or her well-being. For example, if they see the baby's heart rate going down, they will want to figure out the cause immediately. All eyes are constantly watching that fetal monitor for signs of stress. If the baby is in distress, it may necessitate an immediate delivery or C-section.

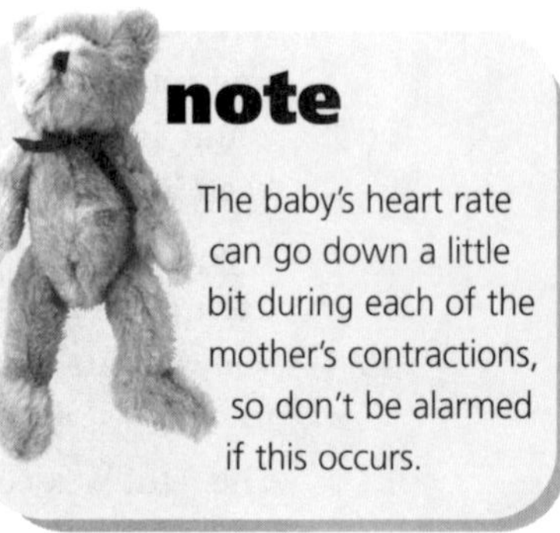

note

The baby's heart rate can go down a little bit during each of the mother's contractions, so don't be alarmed if this occurs.

Questions You'll Be Asked

At this point in your labor, the doctor will take over from the nurse and evaluate your condition. You'll be asked a number of questions, including the following: (I've included my thoughts on these questions in parentheses—sometimes, you just want to kill the hospital staff when you're in labor.)

1. What is your chief complaint, or what brought you in today? (Like, duh! Resist the urge to tell the doctor or nurse to go jump. She truly needs to know if you're in pain and how much.)
2. How many contractions are you having in an hour? (I told you they'd ask this question.)
3. How long are they lasting? (Told ya this as well, so you might as well be prepared and pull out your handy-dandy sheet, thereby blowing them away with your preparation. You need something to give you the upper hand at a time like this!)
4. Are you leaking any fluid? Did your bag of water break? (If the answer is "My God, I hope not," it didn't. You'll know if it breaks—the big gush of water similar to Niagara Falls is a telltale sign.) (See Chapter 13.)
5. Are you bleeding? (Can't you tell? Look and see. Oh, you mean when I was at home…)
6. Did you lose your mucous plug? (What is a mucous plug anyway? Oh, you mean that gross thing?) (See Chapter 13.)
7. Are you feeling the baby move around all right? (I can't bloody well feel anything *but* baby at this point.)
8. Are you feeling all right otherwise? Do you have any fever or other illnesses? (Who are they kidding with this question? At this point, you feel nothing but sick. In fact, you've never felt worse.)

Answers to the above Questions (or Why They Are Important)

Believe it or not, the medical personnel do have valid reasons for asking you all these questions. Here is the information they can glean from your answers.

1. The doctor wants to rule out any problems or potential complications that could occur with the labor and delivery. Be very specific about everything that has happened to you thus far.
2. The number of contractions will give them some clue about how close you are to delivery.
3. Again, they will be able to tell if you're close to delivery. Labor and delivery can be straightforward or extremely complicated. The doctor is always looking for any potential signs of problems.
4. Sometimes, you may *think* you've broken your bag of water, but you haven't. You might just have urine leaking out from the pressure, which is normal. When most women break their bag of water, it's an obvious thing. You'll look down and a pool of water will be under you, and you can't do a thing to stop it. However, some women only leak a small amount of fluid when their water breaks. This might occur in cases where the amniotic fluid volume was low before the bag broke, or the baby's head could have sealed off the leakage and most of the fluid is still behind the baby in the uterus. It's important to know if the bag of water has broken because there is an increased risk for infection and there is less fluid cushioning the baby inside the uterus. Usually, if the water has broken, the doctor will deliver the baby within one to two days.

caution

When the bag of water breaks, the wall between the baby and the bacteria in the vagina is removed, and the bacteria can cross over and cause an infection either in the mother or the baby.

5. Bleeding might indicate a problem with the placenta or in most cases, if the bleeding is minor, it could just indicate dilation of the cervix.
6. The mucous plug sort of acts like a loose cork in the neck of a bottle, the neck of the bottle being the cervix in this case. As the cervix dilates or softens, the cork tends to fall out. What does it look like? Doctors say it kind of looks like snot. It's mucousy, thick and/or runny, stringy, and sometimes pink-tinged. Some women mistake it for their bag of water breaking.
7. Usually, there is a perception that the baby is moving around less than it was, which is probably due to the fact that there is less available room for the baby. This is because the amniotic fluid, which keeps the uterus from squeezing the baby too tightly, tends to decrease towards your due date. (See Chapter 11.)

Horrors—If You're *Not* in Labor

After you and the baby have received a thorough evaluation by the doctors and nurses, and it is determined that you are doing fine, but you're not in labor, then you will likely be sent home and given directions as to when to come back. OK, this may be the lowest point in your whole life. All that excitement and phone calls to assorted friends and family for nothing. Go home with your tail between your legs and rest up, because be assured that you'll be going back to the hospital sooner or later.

FROM THE DOCTOR'S PERSPECTIVE...

When I asked John how common false labor was? His response was a hearty laugh and this insightful message, "Pretty *darn* common!" (OK, he used a slightly more forceful expletive.)

Occasionally, if you're just on the verge of going into labor, the doctor may advise you to stay in the hospital and walk for several hours, up and down the hallways, hoping that it will induce labor. Often, physical activity and gravity (and the baby's head bouncing up and down on the cervix) can push a woman over the edge into labor if she is on the verge. After a period of walking, the doctor will recheck your cervix and see if you've made any further progress. If you have, you'll be admitted into the hospital with a diagnosis of labor, and eventually a baby should make its appearance.

FROM A FRUSTRATED MOTHER'S PERSPECTIVE...

I walked for hours once in that scary hospital gown and those stupid pieces of cardboard they call slippers. Up and down the hallway, past the women who were having babies, up and down, talking to the relatives, up and down, with nothing ever happening. I felt like some kind of freak who didn't have enough sense to get the labor going. Needless to say, I was pissed when nothing happened, and I was sent home.

If your cervix hasn't changed, then the medical personnel feel more reassured that you won't deliver in the very near future (i.e., on the highway going home), so they'll send you home. Let's face it—your doctor would feel pretty bad if she turned on the news and found out you'd delivered on the highway. Other factors that may cause a doctor to follow this "walking" procedure are if the patient lives far away (ergo, might not make it back in time) or if she's had several babies in the past (subsequent births tend to go quickly, leaving no time for the drive back and forth).

THE NEED TO CLEAN

There's an old myth that if you clean your house or scrub the floors, you'll go into labor. If you feel like cleaning the house and getting it in order, by all means, go ahead and do so. While some people may say it doesn't work, my experience is that it is a great indicator of an impending birth. Hey, if you don't go into labor, you'll still have a clean house and feel better. No loss there! Mr. Clean would be proud.

If you are sent home, the doctor will advise you to continue monitoring the progress of your labor. Here are a few precautions to watch out for:

- The contractions worsen compared to what they were when you went into the hospital.
- You suspect your bag of water has broken.
- You have any unusual bleeding.
- You have the perception that your baby isn't moving around well.

If any of these conditions occur, call the hospital or your doctor for advice, or simply go back to the hospital. Otherwise, if you're not having any of these symptoms, try to get some rest and be sure to mention your experience to your own doctor at your next appointment (assuming that he wasn't at the hospital).

What to Pack—Just in Case

Packing a suitcase for the hospital is not as tricky as you might think. After all, if all goes well, your stay there will be limited to a day or two. You'll probably be wearing those god-awful gowns most of the time, at least during the labor and delivery, which doesn't leave a lot of room for any other clothes.

For the Mother

First, pack the amenities: personal soap (if you want it), shampoo, toothpaste, toothbrush, makeup, brush, comb, whatever—the things from home that make you feel like yourself. Second, you'll need a gown of some sort, a robe, and slippers (or sandals if you'd prefer) since you will probably be spending one night there, and really, really don't want to wear their version of a nightgown anymore. If you're nursing, make sure that you pack a nursing bra and a gown that is easily opened or accessible to the baby. If you're not nursing, pack a bra that fit you while you were pregnant, making sure that it has lots of support. The milk will still come in, and your breasts will feel very, very heavy.

You'll need some kind of outfit to wear home. Believe it or not, you won't be wearing your favorite prepregnancy clothes when you leave the hospital. Most of that weight will still be with you for a while, so you might want to wear a loose fitting dress or even maternity pants and tops. That will probably rub you the wrong way, because no one wants to wear maternity clothes after delivery; however, ya gotta do what ya gotta do. You need to be clad in something to escape the hospital confines.

For the Baby

Packing for the baby is a lot more fun than packing for you. If you know the sex, you can obviously choose something that is a suitable color (if you put boys in pink, don't be offended when they're mistaken for girls). It's good to have some kind of gown or sleeper set for the baby. The hospital will supply you with diapers until you leave. An undershirt is a necessity, and they're so cute and tiny. Booties are fun. Forget shoes—babies at that age don't do shoes. If the weather is bad, make sure you have the appropriate attire to wrap the baby in (what's that bundling thing called?). It's always good to bring some baby blankets to wrap them up like a baked potato.

Most importantly, take a car seat. You can't take the baby from the hospital without one.

Oh, and don't forget your camera or video cam. By the way, if your husband or significant other is even marginally competent, he can bring anything you've forgotten to the hospital.

THE ABSOLUTE MINIMUM

When your first baby's birth is imminent, every little change in your body becomes a "real" (at least in your mind) symptom of birth to an expectant mother. In truth, there are some pretty decisive ways to tell whether or not you're in labor. If you match any or all of the criteria listed in this chapter, then you should be having a baby fairly soon.

- Both you and your partner should monitor the spacing and regularity of your contractions. Chart them, if at all possible.
- Your doctor will tell you what specific symptoms to watch for, but if you break your water, call your doctor.
- Braxton-Hicks contractions can make a pregnant woman's life hell, just from the confusion they cause. They can feel very, very real. Don't be afraid to go to the hospital to get checked. Better safe than sorry.
- Pack and prepare in advance as much as possible. You won't be thinking of last-minute details when you're in real labor.

PART V

The Delivery & Post Partum

In This Chapter

- How do the nurses and doctors check to see if you're really in labor?
- Defining the jargon you're going to hear while in labor
- Step-by-step through the labor process
- Defining what happens in a normal delivery

16

What to Expect in a Normal Delivery

OK, so you've read Chapter 15 and are convinced that you're in labor. What are you waiting for? Get thee to a hospital— quickly. Don't forget your suitcase. Don't forget your husband (or partner or coach). Don't forget the way to the hospital. Do pass "Go." Do collect $200 (but only if you're playing Monopoly).

WHEN COOL HEADS SHOULD PREVAIL

You might want to try a few dry runs to the hospital. My mother used to tell the story about her brother who upon hearing that his wife was in labor, jumped into the car, threw in the suitcase, and tore off to the hospital...without his wife, who was left standing in the driveway. Fortunately, he realized his mistake early enough to drive back and get her.

At my second birth, the labor went so quickly that my husband became disoriented while driving to the hospital, even though he should have known the route blindfolded. It was a bit foggy, and I was lying down, moaning and groaning, but had to sit up long enough to give him directions to the hospital.

Moral of the story: Try a few dry runs to make sure you know the best possible route to the hospital. Also, know a few side routes in case your normal way is blocked by construction, an accident, or for some other reason (like your driver is dotty).

Stages of Labor

You'll find that the medical community uses a lot of jargon while you're in labor. We'll try to clear up some of what you're likely to hear and what it means throughout this chapter. There are three stages of labor, and you have to go through all three stages to get to the final outcome, aka the baby. The length and duration of these three stages may vary slightly for each woman.

The first stage of labor is when you are actively having contractions and officially diagnosed as being in labor. This can last a few hours or from to 8–14 hours. The first stage of labor is divided into two phases. The latent phase is the first portion of the first stage. This is the slow, drawn out portion that everybody hates (and they're told, "no, you're not in labor, go home.") Active phase is the second portion of the first stage of labor, and this is when the delivery process occurs at a faster rate. Because labor is more predictable at this point and the progress is steady, patients are typically admitted to the hospital once they reach this point.

The second stage of labor occurs when the cervix is maximally dilated (10 centimeters). This is usually when the mother is told she can push. For a first-time mother if she doesn't have an epidural, this second stage of labor can last one to two hours; with an epidural two to three hours (an epidural can slow labor down).

The third stage of labor begins after the baby is delivered until the placenta comes out. This stage can last up to 30 minutes. We'll break down these stages more completely in the sections that follow.

When You're First Admitted to the Hospital: The Preliminary Exam

After you are evaluated in the labor and delivery area and a determination is made that you are indeed in labor, you will be admitted to the hospital. Forms will need to be signed and papers filled out, but the hospital staff is conscious of the fact that you may be otherwise preoccupied (insert primal scream: I'M IN LABOR—LEAVE ME ALONE!). Your partner can help with this part of the administrative process. In fact, he or she is expected to do so, except for any signatures that you may need to provide.

note

In this section, we're referring mostly to doctors doing the preliminary exam, but it could also be a midwife (if you're using one) or a labor and delivery nurse. Actually, in a hospital setting it's pretty common for nurses to do the preliminary exam before the doctor arrives and then to call the doctor with their results. Labor and delivery nurses are well trained and quite good at these assessments, as they do them every day.

From the time that you are admitted, doctors and nurses will be discussing your examination findings, based on the fetal heart rate tracings and contraction patterns. But first things first—you'll be given a preliminary exam, either by a doctor or a nurse.

Your first exam at the hospital will include a cervical exam, where three areas are measured: your dilation, effacement, and the station.

Dilation of the Cervix

The dilation of the cervix is measured in centimeters. During the exam, the doctor basically is trying to decide how dilated (or open) the cervix is. The doctor will place his hand gently (we hope) inside your vagina all the way up to the cervix to feel the presentation of the baby's body part. He should feel the head if all is well. Occasionally, the baby will be breech—that is, the doctor will feel the baby's butt or feet. If this condition is diagnosed, the patient will probably be advised to have a c-section, or the doctor may try to turn the baby to the head-down position.

Dilation can be measured anywhere from 1–10 centimeters, one being the beginning of the dilation process and 10 being fully dilated (i.e., the baby is almost out). If the cervical dilation is approximately 3–4 centimeters or greater and the mother is contracting regularly, then she will usually be diagnosed as being in active labor and will be admitted to labor and delivery (in first stage labor).

Effacement of the Cervix

In most cases, the baby's head is down, so the doctor continues with his exam and measures the effacement of the cervix (or the thinness of the cervix). Effacement is measured in percentages. In a normal, nonlaboring woman the cervix is 3–4 centimeters long, which is 0% effacement. If a woman is in labor, then the cervix thins. As it thins, it starts to stretch and becomes incorporated into the lower part of the uterus. For example, if the doctor determines the cervix is about 2 cm. thick, then the effacement is approximately 50%.

Station of the Cervix

The station of the baby is based on the relative distance of the baby's presenting body part (the head) to the level of the patient's ischial spines. These ischial spines are part of the bony portions of the mother's pelvis that the doctor or nurse can feel during the exam. A station is described as being anywhere on a scale from –5 to +5 with 0 being at the level of the ischial spine. If the baby is at 0 station, then the top of his head is at the level of the ischial spine. If the baby's station is a positive number, that means that the baby has moved farther down the birth canal past the ischial spine (ergo, closer to delivery).

Putting It All Together

Typical doctor lingo for a woman in labor might be something like this: 4 cm. dilated/50% effaced/–1 station. Translation: The cervix is 4 centimeters open. An effacement of 50% means that half of the cervix is thinned out (or the thickness has decreased by half). And –1 refers to the baby's presenting part or head being –1 cm. above the ischial spines.

If you are having regular contractions with the above diagnosis, then you have passed from the latent phase of labor (or the slow portion of the first stage) into the active phase of labor (or the faster portion of the first stage). For a first-time mother, once she has entered the active phase of labor, then the baby usually will be delivered within 8–12 hours, if not sooner. Patients at the active phase of labor are admitted to the hospital because the chance that the baby will deliver within several hours is fairly high, and the doctors and nurses will want to monitor the patient very closely during this time. This is the phase where the mother and baby are at higher risk for potential complications.

Admission

Once you are officially admitted and taken to a labor and delivery room, the nursing staff will go over certain items with you. They will ask you questions, some of which you may have answered already at your doctor's visits. For example, they will review your medication history and potential allergies. Your doctor (or a nurse) will explain what happens during labor and delivery, if he has not already done so, and go over potential procedures that may or may not need to be performed. Once you have an understanding of what will happen, you will sign a patient consent form, which implies that you understand what will occur in labor and delivery. This time is also your opportunity to ask questions.

A CHANCE FOR PARTNERS TO EARN THEIR KEEP

During this process of admission, you are going to be distracted by contractions and not at your best or sharpest mentally. Your entire focus is on your body and the impending birth of your baby. It's important that your husband, partner, significant other, or coach be alert and attuned to what the nursing staff is explaining. If you don't fully understand what is going on or what the staff is saying, that's OK. Perhaps your partner can explain it to you later. Rely on your partner to go back to the doctor or nurse and get a more satisfactory or fuller explanation, if necessary.

Another tip: You might want to have your partner take a notebook so that he or she can jot down your questions. Or you could prepare some questions in advance. The important thing to remember is that your partner is your advocate. Make sure that person realizes his or her role in your delivery process and just how valuable that role is. (On the other hand, don't let them be too obnoxious, constantly pestering the medical staff and diverting attention from you—it does happen occasionally.)

The question and answer period serves as a protective mechanism for both the hospital and the patient. Some topics that might be discussed with you are the possibility of using forceps, having an episiotomy, what conditions might warrant a c-section, and so on. The patient is protected by virtue of the fact that she knows what is going to happen before it happens (in the best of all possible cases). The hospital and medical staff are protected because they have proof that they told the patient what they were going to do in order to take care of her.

Labor Is Truly Labor-Intensive

Once all the paperwork is done, you'll be admitted to a labor and delivery room, which is usually a private room in most hospitals (although there are exceptions).

An IV (intravenous) line will be placed in one of your arms. This IV line serves multiple purposes:

- Fluids and medications can be administered to the patient while she is in labor.
- Blood transfusions, if needed, can be administered quickly through the IV.
- Pain medications can be administered through the IV, and an anesthesiologist will want to make sure that you have a working IV in case you have an emergency c-section.

SHAVING

As far as shaving the pelvic area, it isn't usually done anymore. The exception might be if the patient undergoes a c-section, in which case the patient might be shaven (depending on the physician's preference). Although shaving was a routine procedure many years ago, the thought process today is that when you shave someone with a razor, you might cut the skin and open up a potential site for infection.

The baby will be placed on an external fetal monitor where the baby's heart rate and the mother's contraction pattern will be evaluated. The mother will also have her blood pressure checked regularly throughout labor. The mother's heart rate can also be monitored with a pulse oximeter, which measures the maternal heart rate, in addition to how well she is oxygenating.

During this time, the doctors and nursing staff will be monitoring the progression or lack of progression of the labor. The doctor will probably check your cervix every two hours, as needed, to determine whether or not you are making progress with cervical dilation, effacement, and station.

The Nurse's Role during Labor

The nurse who is handling your case quickly becomes your best friend in crime, so to speak, because he/she is probably going to be the person whom you see the majority of the time. Usually, the nurse has one-on-one care of a patient, or at most, she might be taking care of two patients at the same time.

The nurse will be your most visible health care provider during the laboring stage. She (or he) attends to your every need, monitors your condition constantly, answers questions, takes care of unwanted visitors, coordinates with the doctor, administers medicines as necessary, listens to your fears, and generally serves as your point man/woman for any problems during your labor. She will check your vital signs, help you go to the bathroom, maintain close observation of the baby's heart rate, and do the necessary charting. She will maintain your IVs. The nurse is there to look out for your best interests. She's also making sure that your spouse and other family members are comfortable as well; but her primary care rests with you, her patient.

Treat this person like gold—they are certifiable saints.

The Doctor's Role during Labor

If you have an outside doctor (meaning he doesn't work at the hospital), he will be notified the moment you arrive and he may ask a nurse to do the initial evaluation. He will immediately make plans to be there for the delivery, but he might not be there for the duration of the labor. Instead, he may ask the nurse to do the cervical check if you're not close to delivery, and then he might ask the nurse to give him a call once the patient reaches 8–10 centimeters. That way, he can complete his schedule with his patients in his office or finish surgery if he's in the middle of surgery. However, if there is a problem, he will drop everything to get there immediately. If the doctor's schedule is free, he will probably go into the hospital to monitor your progress once you're admitted.

When the doctor arrives at the hospital, he will be meeting with you to evaluate your progress and answer any questions. He'll continue to be in touch with your nurse and give orders to the nurse about procedures that need to be given. Even though your doctor may not be in the room as much as your nurse (he may have other patients in the hospital that he's responsible for), he will be accessible and usually waits in the boardroom, which is a place where electronic monitors are centralized. He will be monitoring your heart rate, your contractions, and your baby's heart rate from that remote location within the hospital. If everything is going smoothly with your labor, you will see the doctor every two hours until you are about to deliver. However, if there are any concerns or any problems arise, then the doctor will be coming in more frequently.

Pain Medications during Labor

Labor hurts—no ifs, ands, or buts about it. Once you are in active labor, the pain can be quite significant. But not all women experience the same reaction or level of discomfort with their contractions. If you request pain relief (and don't hesitate to do so if you need it), your doctor will review several options for you, including IV pain medications or regional anesthesia, which can include an epidural or an intrathecal (slightly different location than an epidural). The doctor will determine which one of these regional anesthetics will work best for you. This is not a choice made by the patient. Usually, the doctor will make the choice in consultation with an anesthesiologist.

The IV pain meds are given by the attending physician or nurse. An anesthesiologist usually administers epidurals or regional anesthesia, although your obstetrician may also administer anesthesia, depending on the hospital.

If Your Labor Slows Down, or The Three Ps

Occasionally, the mother's labor pattern may slow down or stall altogether. This could be due to several reasons. First, the contraction pattern may have stopped for an unknown reason also known as a *dysfunctional labor pattern*. Second, the mother may have an infection of the uterus. Third, the mother may not have a pelvis that is the optimal size for a vaginal delivery. In this case, even if the baby is a normal size, it might get hung up on the bony structures within the birth canal. Doctors will check you carefully if your labor slows or stops to try to determine what is going on (or not).

note

Blood work is drawn from the patient and includes ACBC and blood type, meaning that blood is typed and screened. The blood bank is notified so they can be prepared for a cross-match if the patient needs a transfusion. That way compatible blood is available, if necessary.

Typically, doctors check for the three "Ps" when trying to determine why labor has slowed or stopped. The first P refers to power—that is, the frequency, strength, and duration of the contractions. The next P refers to the pelvis. Doctors check to see if the pelvis is large enough for the baby to traverse through it or if there are any obstructions preventing the baby from going through. The third P refers to the passenger (or the baby). Is the baby's size or the way the baby is orienting itself in the pelvis the problem? For example, the head could be down, but turned in an improper way.

In truth, it's usually varying combinations of the three Ps that contribute to protracted or slow labor. The doctor will make the determination as to why the labor has slowed and how best to correct the situation.

INTERNAL MONITORS ON THE BABY

For most patients, external monitors are adequate; however, if the baby's heart rate becomes worrisome or if it's difficult to tell how well a patient is contracting, internal monitors may be recommended. A fetal scalp electrode is placed on the baby's head to measure the baby's heart rate and any abnormalities. There might also be an IUPC (intrauterine pressure catheter) inserted that is not attached to the baby, but is a flexible probe inserted between the baby and the uterine wall through the vagina. This device detects the strength of the contractions and offers a more accurate interpretation of labor. The IUPC also serves as a means to increase the amount of fluid surrounding the baby, called an amnio infusion. This occurs when saline or water is transfused into the space around the baby and provides additional cushioning for the umbilical cord in times of stress. When the patient gets internal monitors, the external monitors are removed. There is a slightly increased chance of infection, which is why these monitors aren't routinely placed on all patients.

Using Pitocin to Speed Up Labor

If your labor has slowed or stopped and the doctor has made the assessment of the three Ps and it is still possible to deliver vaginally, then the doctor might administer pitocin through an IV. Pitocin is a medicine that stimulates the uterus to contract. It mimics the body's own natural hormone called *oxytocin*, which is supposed to do the same thing—that is, speed up labor. Pitocin is generally a safe medicine; however, there are some precautions that need to be taken—for example, its dosage needs to be carefully regulated.

In rare circumstances, the uterus may become overstimulated, in which case the uterus contracts so frequently that the baby receives less oxygen. This may lead to a decrease in the baby's heart rate as the uterus doesn't have any downtime from the contractions. When the uterus is contracting, oxygen is at its worst for the baby. During the relaxation phase between contractions, the baby's optimal oxygen status is usually restored.

If, by some chance, the contractions become too frequent, the doctors will recommend turning down or turning off the pitocin temporarily in order to give the baby a break and a chance to recover sufficiently. In extreme circumstances, when this does not work, the doctor may recommend that the patient receive a different medication to relax the uterus and counteract the effects of pitocin temporarily.

One other potential complication from pitocin is that the uterus could rupture, due to hyperstimulation (overstimulation) or extreme contraction strength generated by the drug.

For these reasons, the drug is carefully monitored at all times.

Repositioning the Baby

If the doctor determines that your lack of progress is due to the baby's position or malpresentation, then the doctor may attempt to reposition the baby's head during a vaginal exam, if at all possible. To do this, the doctor will gently feel the landmarks on the baby's skull to imagine which way the baby's head is pointed. Then he will attempt to turn the baby and correct any malpresentation that exists.

Many times, labor will resume in a normal fashion after repositioning without any further intervention, and the mother will eventually reach maximal dilation of 10 centimeters. When the mother is maximally dilated and effacement is 100%, then she is ready to push.

Pushing and Delivery

Usually, the patient's nurse or doctor will have coached her ahead of time so that she knows what to expect when they ask her to push. Pushing is timed to coincide with each contraction for maximum effect. When the uterus is contracting, this is the best time for the mother to exert her pushing efforts in order to deliver the baby. A contraction lasts approximately one minute. She will be asked to push three times during each contraction, with each effort lasting approximately 10 seconds.

Pushing

In-between contractions, the patient is asked to rest and not push, but to take slow deep breaths of oxygen in order to give the baby as much oxygen as possible. Remember, this is one of the most stressful times for the baby. Not only is the uterus contracting, but most of the amniotic fluid has leaked out so there is less cushioning to counteract the pressure that is being generated by the contracting uterus. Also, the space is tighter for the baby as it works its way down the birth canal.

In the early stages of pushing, the doctor or nurse may be examining you simultaneously with your pushing. For the doctor, this is a good opportunity to see how effective the patient is able to push.

FROM THE DOCTOR'S PERSPECTIVE...

I always ask my patient to pay close attention to my assessment of how well she is pushing while I'm examining her. I want her to focus on those pushing efforts that I've found to be effective and that are allowing her to progress, and for her to continue focusing on that particular pushing effort that she has made with each successive contraction. I'm providing her with feedback as to how well she is doing so that she can minimize any wasted effort and deliver the baby successfully.

There is the potential for the mother to tire out very quickly, so I don't want her to push in an ineffective way if at all possible. In between contractions, I advise patients to remember what they did right so they won't start the next contraction without knowing how to push effectively. I'm examining the baby's head while the mother is pushing so that I can tell if the baby is rotating or coming down the birth canal properly. Unfortunately, there is the potential for the mother to become distracted by her family with oohs and aahs of excitement. I want her to stay on track and not lose focus.

FROM THE MOTHER'S PERSPECTIVE...

Hey, I delivered five times, and each time I was clueless about what an effective push was and what wasn't. They all felt the same. First of all, it's difficult to tell if you're pushing or not, since what constitutes "pushing" doesn't make a lot of sense. Second, when you're at that phase, it's all a blur. Your only thought is "GET THIS BABY OUT OF ME!" and do whatever it takes. Sorry, Dr. John. Maybe if you'd been my doctor I would have known what an effective push was.

What Everyone Else Is Doing While You're Pushing (aside from Taking Bets)

The doctor will usually have the spouse of the patient get involved in the labor and delivery process. The spouse will stand on the opposite side of where the nurse is, supporting the patient both emotionally and physically while she's pushing (her chin will be pressed against her chest). The patient is asked to open her legs as wide as possible, so the spouse can support her neck and legs on one side, while the nurse supports the other side (picture Twister on a Saturday night). In between contractions the spouse will encourage the patient with words, wipe her forehead with a cool towel, and feed her ice chips if necessary, providing basic support to help the mother deliver the baby.

The nurse is continually monitoring the baby's heart rate and checking the mother's blood pressure. She is also ensuring that IV fluids are running and not stopped for any reason and that drugs or medicines are being administered. The nurse has a huge responsibility during this time, as she is also charting everything that occurs and assisting the doctor as necessary. If requested by the patient, the nurse will bring in a mirror to position between the mother's legs so that she can watch her baby's head as it appears. Some mothers close their eyes through the whole pushing effort, while others may choose to see everything. According to Dr. John, to doctors it is a beautiful experience, but the mother may or may not share that sentiment.

The Delivery

When it's time for the baby's head to deliver, the doctor will do his best to protect the delivery of the head and the mother's perineum to reduce or minimize any tears that might occur. Once the baby's head is delivered, the doctor will ask the mother to stop pushing temporarily. He will suction the mouth and nose of the baby, removing mucous secretion and amniotic fluid that may be present. He will check around the baby's neck to make sure the umbilical cord isn't wrapped around it. If it is, depending on how loose it is, he may unwrap the cord around the baby's neck. Sometimes, the cord may be tightly wrapped around the baby's neck; in that event, the doctor will clamp the cord in two places, cut the cord in-between the two clamps, unwrap the cord manually, and deliver the rest of the baby.

It's a wonderful time for the mother to watch as her entire baby is delivered. Many times a large amount of amniotic fluid that was behind the baby will now flow out. The doctor will also maintain support of the perineum so that there is a minimal chance of tearing. After the baby is delivered, the umbilical cord will be clamped and cut. If the father is interested, he can be given the opportunity to cut the cord. Again, this is a great way of making the extra person feel included in the process.

The baby will be gently stimulated by the delivering doctor and may be placed on the mother's chest or belly and covered with a blanket to provide warmth. The mother is asked to gently stimulate the baby during this time by rubbing the baby's back. Alternatively, the baby may be transferred to the baby warmer station where the medical staff will clean him, warm him, and check his heart rate. If the baby is not doing well, then there may not be time for him to go to his mother. Out of medical necessity, in this case, the baby will go immediately to the warmer or the nursery.

After the baby is born, the doctor and nurse return their attention to their primary patient, the mother. The doctor will reassess the mother's physical status, vital signs will be checked, and the amount of bleeding from the vagina will be determined. The doctor will assess his patient for tears or lacerations that might have occurred in the perineum or vagina or vulva. If any repairs are necessary, the doctor may proceed to do the repairs or opt to do them after the placenta is delivered. The doctor will also see if the cervix has any tears or lacerations, as well as examining the rectum for tears.

If there are any tears from a natural occurrence or from an episiotomy, the doctor will stitch the tears with absorbable sutures, meaning that the suture material will degrade on its own based on the body's ability to break down the suture.

The placenta will be delivered within half an hour after the baby's birth. After the delivery, there is a tendency for the uterus to squeeze down upon itself and return to a contracted state. The placenta will begin to sheer off with the contractions. As it sheers off, there is usually a visible sign of this by a large amount of blood coming out of the vagina and the umbilical cord will lengthen and advance out.

The doctor may aid this process by gentle traction (pulling), but he must be careful not to exert any unnecessary traction, as it could tear the cord off. After the placenta is delivered, the doctor will check to make sure that all of it is intact and no pieces remain in the uterus (which could cause bleeding and infection). The doctor will advise the nurse that the placenta has been delivered, so that she can note the time.

He will ask for pitocin to be administered intravenously, which aids in the contraction of the uterus and stops bleeding. To aid this process, the doctor will massage the uterus and stimulate it physically. The doctor will then check for any remaining clots before the placenta was delivered and evacuate those as necessary. Once the bleeding is under control and all lacerations have been repaired, the patient can be cleaned and her bed will be put back together. She can begin to rest. This is still a potentially dangerous time for the mother as bleeding may resume, so the nurse will continue to check her vital signs (including blood pressure) for the next several hours. The nurse will also check the uterus by pushing down on the abdomen, to make sure that the uterus is contracted and firm to touch. A soft, boggy or enlarged uterus could indicate that bleeding has occurred and the uterus is expanding with blood. That condition may necessitate additional measures, such as checking for clots remaining inside the vagina and uterus, recommendation for additional medications, and a possible blood transfusion. And if bleeding is extreme, surgical measures may be recommended, such as a D & C or a full hysterectomy.

Episiotomy

Often the baby may not be delivered because the vaginal opening is too small or constricted. At other times, the vaginal opening may be appropriate in size, but it has not had enough time to stretch for the baby. Or the baby's heart rate may be of concern to the doctor, so an attempt to expedite delivery may occur. These are all good examples of why an episiotomy might need to be performed.

An episiotomy is a process by which a doctor will make an incision or cut in the space between the vagina and rectum in order to expand the opening for the baby's head. Most doctors do not do this routinely, but rather only when a medical indication arises. When the doctor makes the cut, the vaginal space is enlarged. Of course, after the baby is delivered, the incision or episiotomy must be repaired to restore it to its original anatomy. Occasionally, the episiotomy may be so extensive that it extends to the rectal area. Obviously, this will necessitate more extensive repair afterwards.

Forceps or a Vacuum

In rare circumstances, your baby may need to be delivered with the aid of forceps or a vacuum device. The concept of doing an instrumented vaginal delivery is not new. Forceps have been utilized over the centuries, and they can provide a means to assist in the delivery of a baby when certain conditions arise. For example, if a mother is too tired to push or if the fetal heart rate becomes worrisome, then conditions may warrant the use of forceps or a vacuum. Very strict criteria need to be met before the use of these instruments can be offered to the patient.

If the doctor thinks the conditions are ideal for an instrumented vaginal delivery, then he should discuss his thoughts with the patient so the patient understands the indications, risks, and benefits. Unfortunately, sometimes there isn't time to have a lengthy discussion when the baby's life is at stake, so it's good to go over these procedures with your doctor in advance of the delivery.

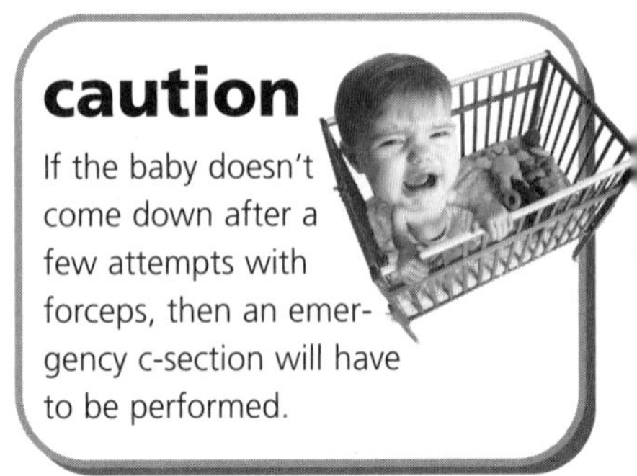

caution

If the baby doesn't come down after a few attempts with forceps, then an emergency c-section will have to be performed.

The benefit to these two procedures is obvious: They may assist in getting the baby out quickly when there is a fetal heartrate problem.

The risks of using either vacuum or forceps are also obvious. They include the potential to injure the baby and create vaginal tears in the mother. You may see slight bruising of the side of the head on a baby where forceps were used. This bruising usually goes away in a few days.

The choice between using a vacuum or forceps is up to the doctor, depending on the patient's condition. The clinical situation will dictate which instrument is chosen. Safety for both the patient and the baby is of utmost importance.

THE ABSOLUTE MINIMUM

A normal delivery is never really normal, simply because it's yours, and that makes it special. However, many of the procedures that you will encounter are easily decipherable and predictable if you simply do your homework in advance.

- Try to study and recognize the phases and stages of labor so you know where you are in the process. Make sure that your partner is equally well informed.
- Pay attention to what the doctors and nurses say to you. Often, they are asking for or giving you information that will expedite your delivery.
- Don't allow too many people into the labor and delivery room with you. Remember—you're there to do a job—deliver your baby. Doing that job requires your full attention and focus. The baby's health is at stake, as is yours.
- When it's all finished, take a moment to bask in what you've accomplished. You've just delivered a new life into the world. Congratulations! It's a miracle each and every time.

IN THIS CHAPTER

- Defining a c-section as opposed to a vaginal birth
- When is a c-section necessary?
- Are elective c-sections an option?
- What happens during a c-section?
- What to expect in recovery and post-op

17

WHAT TO EXPECT IN A C-SECTION

The origin of the term "cesarean section" (more commonly known as a *c-section*) is unknown, although there is much speculation that the name was derived from Julius Caesar, who was thought to be the first live infant born by this method (in 100 B.C.). However, most scholars believe this to be untrue since Caesar's mother lived to a ripe old age; and, typically, many cesarean sections performed before 1930 (when antibiotics were created) resulted in the death of the mother.

Let's start by defining a c-section. A vaginal delivery occurs when the baby is delivered through the vagina by natural means. In a c-section the baby does not go through the birth canal, but rather is pulled out through an incision made in the mother's abdomen and uterus. Unlike a vaginal delivery, a c-section involves a surgical procedure and is performed in an operating room under sterile conditions.

In the United States, approximately one in four babies is delivered by c-section, according to the American College of Obstetricians and Gynecologists (see Figure 17.1).

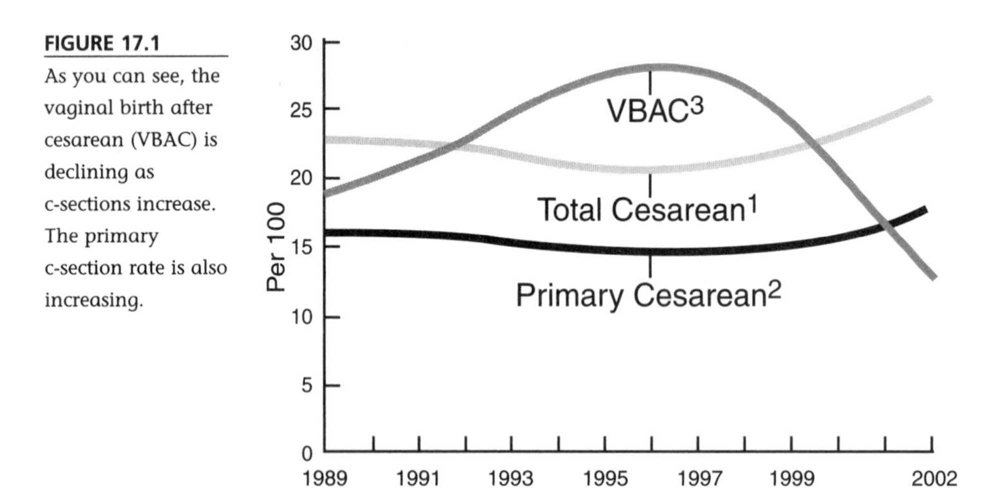

FIGURE 17.1

As you can see, the vaginal birth after cesarean (VBAC) is declining as c-sections increase. The primary c-section rate is also increasing.

When to Perform a C-Section

It's important to note that, in most cases, doctors will opt for a vaginal delivery over a c-section. The reason is that a vaginal delivery is almost always considered to be safer for the mother and baby unless extreme health conditions warrant otherwise. C-sections may be scheduled in advance if certain conditions are present and both the mother and doctor agree that it is necessary.

Often, however, c-sections are performed in emergency circumstances because conditions indicate that the mother or baby is at risk for a potential problem. If the mother's or baby's health is at risk, then a c-section might become the immediate alternative for saving lives. So, you may go into the delivery room anticipating a "normal" delivery and suddenly find that you're going to have a c-section. It's impossible to tell when this will occur, but some of the circumstances that might precipitate this decision on the part of your doctor are listed below.

Maternal Indications for a C-Section

There are several conditions in the mother that would necessitate a c-section (or in doctor jargon, absolute indications—in other words, the doctor would always suggest or resort to a c-section in these cases). If these conditions are noted in advance, chances are good that you'll be scheduled for a c-section when your baby is at term. These health conditions include the following:

- A woman who cannot labor for various reasons (for example, she has a serious heart condition).
- A woman who has a small or contracted pelvis that wouldn't allow the baby to push through (sometimes this is known in advance, but not always).
- Serious maternal health problems where a delivery through the vaginal area would put the baby at risk (for example, the mother has herpes or AIDs).
- If the mother has had a prior classical c-section in a previous birth.

Fetal Indications for a C-Section

In addition, there are conditions related to the baby's health that would prompt the doctor to suggest a c-section over a vaginal delivery. These conditions may not be known in advance of the baby's birth. They include the following:

- Problems with the umbilical cord; for example, the cord falls into the vagina (prolapsed cord, which would lead to emergency surgery) or the cord is pinched or compressed.
- Presence of a complete placenta previa (where the placenta is covering the cervix).
- Fetal distress—that is, the baby shows signs of distress such as a slowing heart rate or lactic acid buildup in the baby's bloodstream from lack of oxygen.
- Fetal illness, which might include babies diagnosed prenatally with certain medical conditions, such as a heart condition or spina bifida (a hole in the spinal cord).
- Multiple babies—that is, twins, triplets, or more.

Possible But Not Absolute Indicators for a C-Section

Then there are conditions that occur where the doctor has the option for a c-section, but may or may not decide to perform one. These are the cases where it helps to trust your doctors and have confidence in their decisions. Remember, these conditions can go either way—meaning, the doctor may or may not decide to perform a c-section, but one could be warranted. Make sure your doctor discusses it with you or your partner first. (However, if the condition is life threatening, there may not be enough time.) These conditions include the following:

- Bleeding from the placenta
- Delivery is advisable immediately, but the mother is not in labor (reasons could include infection or severe preeclampsia)
- Water breaks but no indication of labor and 24 hours have passed
- Shoulder or breech presentation of the baby (the baby's buttocks or feet enter the canal first, instead of the head)
- More than one baby (many women having twins are able to deliver vaginally, but the risk for problems increases with the number of babies)
- Failure of labor to progress in a timely fashion
- Abnormal pelvic structure in the mother (for example, if the mother has had an injury to the pelvis or was born with a pelvic defect)
- If the mother has had a prior low-transverse c-section in a previous birth (see section entitled "Low-Transverse C-Section" later in this chapter for more information)

note

The American College of Obstetrics and Gynecology advises that if the baby is over 11 pounds (5,000 grams), the doctor may advise the woman to have a c-section. However, estimating fetal weight is an inaccurate science in the late third trimester because it's difficult to get accurate measurements using an ultrasound. So doctors do the best they can. The 5,000-gram estimate takes into account a 20% possible discrepancy between the estimated weight and the actual fetal weight.

Elective C-Sections (for the Convenience of the Patient)

Having a c-section just because it's more convenient (meaning you can schedule your child's birth) is a very controversial issue today, especially for first-time mothers. It's especially controversial if there are no known maternal or fetal issues indicating that the c-section is necessary. Traditionally, the thought process was that c-sections were riskier for both mother and baby compared to vaginal deliveries. Traditionalists say that c-sections put the mother at risk unnecessarily, and doctors and patients alike have to deal with the problems of repeat c-sections, which are not a trivial matter.

Proponents of voluntary c-sections argue that it is a woman's right to choose her type of delivery option and that even though the risk is increased, the overall risk is low. According to Dr. John, this is not a settled issue in the OB field, but it is being addressed in various forms, both from the patient safety standpoint and also from an ethical, moral standpoint.

Dr. John feels that it is helpful to address the reasons why the patient might want a c-section when discussing elective surgery. He's found that often the reason might be related to the patient's fears—the fear of unknown pain that might be experienced in labor being the most common. In counseling the patient and addressing the pain issue, Dr. John's patients have usually reconsidered having an elective c-section and opted for a vaginal delivery instead. "I've never had to do an elective primary c-section after I talked to my patient and relieved her concerns," he said.

caution

There is a growing movement in the U.S. to have elective primary c-sections, meaning that women can choose to have a c-section for her *first* delivery instead of a vaginal delivery. This is even more prevalent in other areas of the world, for example, Brazil has an 80% rate of c-sections, while in Italy it is 40%. Why the change? While no one knows the exact answer, there is much speculation.

Some reasons cited are fear of labor; fear of pain that is unable to be addressed; concern that a vaginal delivery will lead to urinary incontinence in later years from overstretching; psychological issues; or convenience and scheduling issues for the doctor or patient.

Or it might be as simple as a patient control issue—a woman wants to have her baby a certain week because her in-laws have plane tickets for that week. Keep in mind that your convenience for the delivery date is *not* more important than your health or your baby's health. The risks of C-sections when compared to vaginal deliveries are much higher and potentially subject the mother and the baby to more problems. For example, there is twice the risk of infection; twice the risk of bleeding compared to vaginal delivery; and an increased risk of a thrombo-embolism (blood clot).

What Is a Classical C-Section?

The classical c-section has been used by physicians as the standard way of performing a c-section, but recently it has been superceded in use by the Low-Transverse uterine incision (see next section).

In a classical c-section, the physician makes an incision or cut in the upper or contractile portion of the uterus. This gives much more access to the baby. It traditionally has been done under emergency circumstances, so many doctors thought this was the quickest and easiest way to deliver the baby. However, as doctors discovered later, this type of incision subjected both the mother and baby to additional risks, as will be discussed later.

While we're on the subject, don't confuse the way your skin is cut and the way your uterus is cut. We're talking about the cutting of the uterus here, not the incision in the skin that you see—confusing, but important differences. Just because a doctor cuts your outer skin up and down or a bikini cut (sideways) doesn't mean that he cuts your uterus that same way. You can't tell from the outer skin incision how your uterus was cut, and it does matter later if you plan on having subsequent births.

The old dictum was once a C-section, always a C-section, which usually applied to the classical Cesarean section and meant that you always had to have C-sections for later deliveries. However, that dictum does not always apply to a low-transverse C-section.

Risks of a Classical C-Section

When a classical C-section is performed, the area that is cut tends to be muscular so that when a scar forms, the scar is found to be weaker when laboring with a future pregnancy. This does not bode well for a mother's attempt at a vaginal delivery in subsequent births, for fear that the scar might tear while in labor. Thus, there is a risk in future deliveries for the uterus to rupture.

If a rupture occurs, the mother could bleed internally, and the baby could work its way through the previous incision or scar. In that case, the placenta would be compromised, and the baby could die. The mother could also die. The overall risk of a uterine rupture occurring is less than one percent in women who have never had surgery of the uterus (for example, a previous baby born by this type of C-section).

However, in women who have had a classical C-section in a previous birth, the risk for rupture elevates to 20-25 percent in subsequent pregnancies and births attempted vaginally. For this reason, most doctors recommend that subsequent births also be delivered via C-section.

In contrast, the risk for rupture in subsequent pregnancies for a woman with one low-transverse C-section is less than one percent. And that's the real reason that OBs prefer the low-transverse c-section procedure.

UNCOVERING STATISTICS

How did doctors figure this out? Dr. John said that there is an unfounded story that the difference between these two types of c-sections in subsequent births was first noticed in the UCLA parking lot, of all places! One day the parking lot was literally full of women having babies at the County Hospital because the hospital was full, and there weren't enough rooms. Because many of the women were Hispanic and possibly there weren't enough interpreters or time to get full histories or data before the births, it wasn't until after the births occurred that doctors discovered that many of the women were having a third or fourth child delivered vaginally, but they had previously had low-transverse incisions and c-sections. Bells started ringing and people started asking questions. The result: The discovery that low-transverse incisions are safer for vaginal deliveries after c-sections. (Hey, it's a good story whether it's true or not.)

Low Transverse C-Section

In a low transverse C-section (LTCS), the doctor cuts through the lower uterine segment of the uterus, which typically doesn't involve the same tissue as a classical C-section. This region of the uterus has less muscular fiber, and is less easy to tear or rupture with future labors.

> **note**
>
> Again, remember that a uterine incision is not the skin incision that you see on your body. The uterine incision is inside of you.

There are still risks with a LTCS, but they seem to be fewer in nature. The uterine scar will tear less easily, as we already suggested. However, even though many women can deliver subsequent babies vaginally after this procedure, many doctors still advise going the C-section route with subsequent babies, just to be on the safe side.

What Happens During a Planned C-section?

In a planned C-section (make note of the word "planned" because procedures might work differently in an emergency), the doctor will review the patient's history, make recommendations, and schedule a certain day and time for the surgery.

Before the Surgery

On the day prior to the surgery, the patient is asked not to eat or drink anything after midnight because she should ideally have an empty stomach in order to keep from aspirating. Aspiration occurs when the patient vomits the contents of her stomach, the contents go back into her throat, and then possibly fall back down the windpipe and into her lungs. This is obviously not a good thing and could be life-threatening. The doctor will ask the patient to show up at the hospital at a specific time. (Dr. John stresses how important it is to be on time. Even though it is several hours before your surgery, there is a lot of prep work that has to be done.) The patient will also be informed of any requisite postoperative restrictions, as well as ensuring that she has adequate help after the surgery.

> **note**
>
> In a perfect world, typically beforehand (either in the doctor's office or prior to surgery), the patient will also receive a counseling session regarding the risks and benefits of c-sections, as well as alternatives.

Pre-Surgery

On the morning of the surgery, the nurse will evaluate the baby's heart rate and mother's contraction pattern by using external monitors placed around the mother's abdomen. In addition, the nurse will check the mother's vital signs. The nurse, doctor, and anesthesiologist will review the records again to evaluate any medical complications. Consent forms will be signed and witnessed. The surgeon will ask the mother if she has any questions and will explain what will happen, if that has not already occurred.

Once everything is set, the patient will be taken to the operating room (OR). The nurse may or may not do a shave of the pubic area, depending on the physician's preference. A Foley bladder catheter is inserted to drain the bladder so that it is not in the way of the operating field (basically, they deflate it). At this point, the anesthesiologist takes over. If the indication is not urgent, the patient will receive a regional anesthetic (most likely a spinal) so she stays awake, but the region being worked on is numb. In this way, the patient does not have to be intubated as she is breathing on her own. This is considered to be much safer than a general anesthetic where the patient is put under and is not conscious. (Much nicer to be conscious for your baby's birth.)

If the baby has been continuously monitored up to this point, the monitors are taken away so that the abdomen can be prepared for surgery. The preparation consists of applying sterilizing solutions to kill all the germs on the surface of the skin. Many times it is an iodine solution. If you're allergic to iodine, let the doctor know earlier. Also, let them know if you're allergic to latex.

Before the surgery begins, a hip roll is placed beneath the patient's right hip, to tilt her slightly to the left. They do this for the same reason that the doctors don't want you sleeping on your back during the latter stages of pregnancy—because the uterus being heavy can rest on the vena cava, which can restrict the blood flow to the baby.

The patient is then draped, and the surgeons take their places on either side of the patient. Often,

tip

You might hear the doctor ask the anesthesiologist "Is Allis home?", leading you to believe if you're the patient that you are truly sedated or going nuts. This is a joke among doctors. (Hey, no one ever called them comedians or insinuated they were highly imaginative.) The derivation of the joke is simple. "Allis" refers to an Allis clamp, which is used to pinch the mother in the area that is being anesthetized. The doctors don't want to ask the patient if she hurts or tip her off in any way that they are testing her for pain, figuring that she will always answer in the affirmative. So, if the anesthesiologist responds that "Allis is home," then the surgeon knows he's good to go. Onward with the operation.

there is a second surgeon (who might be a resident) assisting the primary surgeon (your doctor). Obviously, the primary surgeon will be the person performing the operation.

At this point, the surgeon will check with the anesthesiologist to verify that the anesthesia is adequate—in other words, they will do a test to make sure the patient can't feel anything in the appropriate area and therefore is ready for surgery. Now the father or significant other is allowed into the operating room. That person will be draped in a gown and facemask to preserve the sterile environment, and he (or she) will be positioned at the head of the bed next to you.

The drape is elevated above the patient's chest so that her face is shielded from the operative field. This is done for two reasons: Doctors want to keep the patient's face shielded from anything that could splatter on it; they also don't want her seeing the trauma of her innards coming out. Let's face it—that would be a disgusting thing to witness. So, it's a combination of emotional and physical safety issues.

Surgery

Next, the doctor makes the incision in the skin. Typically, it's called a Pfannenstiel skin incision (otherwise known as a *bikini cut*), which is a horizontal incision just above the pubic hairline. Several layers of tissue are cut before the surgeon is inside reaching the uterus.

From the patient's perspective, all she should feel is a little bit of pressure or tugging and pulling, but she shouldn't feel any sharpness or pain.

After the surgeon reaches the uterus, he will study the anatomy to decide where the baby is lying and where to make the cut to optimize getting the baby out. There will be some gentle dissection behind the bladder in order to create a space to expose the incision site on the uterus. The reason the surgeon takes so much care is that he is trying to preserve the mother's option of having a baby vaginally in the future.

> **caution**
>
> It may seem at first glance that if the incision on your skin is horizontal or transverse, that the cut on your uterus would be the same, but that isn't necessarily the case. Make sure that you get a copy of your medical report because if you switch doctors, your future OB will want to know how your uterus was cut to determine the next pregnancy's delivery method.

The physician will make a low-transverse uterine incision. The incision will be large enough to pull the baby out, possibly 8–10 centimeters (the doctor can stretch it more with his hands). The surgeon will go slowly before the next cut, with the assistant suctioning away the blood that obscures the surgeon's vision. There is lots of blood pouring into the hole he is cutting, so he must trust his tactile feel to reduce injury to the baby. Once the doctor feels that he is inside the uterus, he will stretch open the incision and put one hand inside to protect and deliver the baby's head. Usually, he will be aided by an assistant who is applying pressure on the top of the uterus to push the baby forward.

The baby's head can't be pulled out until it's actually peeking out. The surgeon will use a little force to push the mother's uterus down, thereby squeezing the baby out of the incision.

From the mother's perspective, she'll feel tugging and a lot of pressure. She will *not* be asked to push, but she will definitely be aware of the tugging and pulling.

The Baby Delivered by C-Section

When the baby is delivered, there tends to be a lot of amniotic fluid that comes out, so the doctor will suction the baby's mouth and nose to aid the baby's breathing efforts. He'll clamp the umbilical cord, cut the cord between two clamps, and one of the doctors will hand the baby to a nurse so that the baby can go immediately to a warmer. (The doctor might show you the baby briefly, but don't count on it. The immediate concern is to get the baby evaluated.) After the baby is on the warmer, the neonatal resuscitative team (NNR) will work on the baby and make sure that it is progressing as it should.

The way the staff handles a baby delivered by Cesarean is different than the way they handle a vaginal birth because of the increased risk to both mother and baby in a c-section. For example, the baby may have more of an adjustment or transition period from intrauterine to extrauterine life by being delivered from a c-section. In a vaginal delivery, the squeezing of going through the birth canal pushes the fluid in the baby's lungs out and can facilitate breathing of the baby once it's delivered. However, in a c-section, depending upon whether labor occurred or not, much of this fluid may still remain in the baby's lungs, so the baby is often given oxygen and the baby's back is massaged (palpation) to increase the expulsion of fluid.

The Surgery Continues...

Once the baby is out, the OB will focus his attention back on the mother (his primary patient) because she is still bleeding from the uterus, which must be controlled immediately.

The placenta is delivered next. The surgeon places his hand inside the uterus and peels the placenta off the uterine wall. Simultaneously, the anesthesiologist administers Pitocin, which will help the uterus squeeze down upon itself to cut down on the blood loss. Typically, if the patient hasn't received antibiotics up to this point, she will receive them now. Antibiotics are a key factor because they will reduce the chances of infection, since virtually all the contents of the uterus have spilled into the patient's abdominal cavity , including lots of bacteria (not to be too graphic here, but yeech—I'm beginning to notice that doctors get a kick out of describing gross stuff).

Once the placenta is out, the doctor focuses on closing the incision he made. There tends to be a lot of bleeding at this juncture, so visualization is a challenge. The team uses a combination of suction and gauze sponges to find out where they need to sew. They start at one end of the uterine incision and work across to the other side, closing the incision site. Often, the OB will perform a second layer of closure on top of the first one. Some doctors feel that this is helpful to prevent a uterine rupture in the future.

Next, the surgeon will look for any signs of bleeding that haven't been addressed yet and cauterize those areas. The pelvic region may be irrigated with sterile water or saline. The doctor will remove any large clots and begin the closure of the various layers of incisions that were previously incised, including the skin. The skin may be closed with suture materials or staples.

FROM THE DOCTOR'S PERSPECTIVE...

Studies show that the healing rates from using either staples or suture material are the same. Dr. John, however, likes sutures better because they are dissolvable. "With staples, you have to remove them in three days, say the morning of going home. Sutures don't have to be removed since they dissolve on their own. Some doctors think it's faster to work with staples, but I still prefer sutures."

The Pitfalls of Surgery

Compared to a vaginal delivery, the risk for the mother in a C-section is generally twice that of a vaginal birth for bleeding, infection, and other complications. Having said that, the overall risk of having a complication is one to three percent.

The mother could also have injury to other organs, including the bladder and intestines. In rare cases, the uterus may continue to bleed despite conservative efforts to stop the bleeding. In those situations, it's possible that a hysterectomy might have to be performed. This would be done as a last resort to save a woman's life. The decision is never taken lightly. With any surgery, there is also the risk of scar tissue or adhesions, which could cause pain later.

One of the obvious risks for the baby is that the doctor could cut the baby's skin with the scalpel. Because the baby's head or face is pressed against the uterus, the doctor has to go very slowly and carefully when incising the uterus, clearing away blood before making his every cut. That is where experience and touch come into play for the surgeon, who is often blinded by the extensive amount of blood. Other injuries the baby could suffer might be a neck injury, as it is being pulled out.

Post-Op and Recovery

After the woman is all stitched up, she is transported (referred to as *towed* in the Navy) to the recovery room for at least an hour. There her vital signs are monitored to make sure there are no significant complications from surgery that would require her to go back to the OR. If the baby is doing fine, she may see the baby at this point, or she may have to wait until she goes to her room. Sometimes, it's hard for family members to visit in the recovery room due to privacy issues with other patients, so don't expect a lot of visitors.

Typically, your OB will sit down and explain how the surgery went and answer any questions. Afterwards, the patient is transferred to a recovery room or a postpartum room, where she will stay until she is discharged, which will probably be in two or three days, barring complications.

The Day of the Surgery

The day of the surgery, if you're the patient, you will feel pretty tired and have some pain issues. You will be required to rest a lot. The catheter will stay in place so that you don't have to get out of bed to go to the bathroom. Pain medicines will be administered through an IV. You will not be allowed to eat at first, although fluids are provided. Mostly, you'll just want to rest (and see your baby, of course).

The First Day Post-Op

By the first day after surgery (post-operative Day 1), the doctor will evaluate you to make sure you're stable. The bandage will be removed so the doctor can look at the incision, and then it will be left uncovered. The Foley catheter is removed. The patient is asked to begin walking, if she hasn't already done so.

Walking will be a little bit challenging at first, but with effort, the majority of women find they can walk pretty well by the end of the first day. Dr. John always asks patients to sit up for a few minutes first to make sure they aren't dizzy, and then stand up with a hand close to the bed to give themselves another minute before they walk around the room.

You will still have an IV with fluid flowing. You should sit in a chair if you're tired but don't feel like sleeping. If you're tired, use the bed to sleep, but if you're not tired, doctors prefer that you try to use the chair. Sitting and walking not only restores confidence, but also helps prevent clots from forming in the legs. You'll be asked to increase your walking daily.

It's time for food, if you feel like eating. The first meal you will eat will be a soft diet of easily chewed foods. If those are tolerated well, you'll advance to eating regular foods.

The Second Day Post-Op

On the second day, the hospital staff and your doctor will evaluate your progress and take a blood test to make sure you haven't lost too much blood. You'll continue to walk the hallways, obviously more than the day before. In some instances, patients may recover so well that they can be discharged at the end of the day, but this is usually reserved for post-op Day 3.

The Third Day Post-Op

On post-op Day 3, you'll be examined, the staples will be removed if necessary, and you'll be given instructions on how to take care of yourself at home. Things to watch out for include fevers, increased vaginal bleeding (more than a period), and pain that is not responding to pain meds that could indicate complications from surgery. The doctor will recommend that you don't lift anything heavier than your baby.

Home Care

For six weeks, you should watch for all of the above (fever, vaginal bleeding, and pain), but precautions also should include not placing anything inside the vagina (this means no tampons, douching, or sexual intercourse). Some doctors recommend driving restrictions (meaning don't drive) from three to four weeks or longer.

> **tip**
>
> Be sure to check with your auto insurance company about this restriction, because in rare cases, your insurance might have its own restrictions regarding surgery limitations.

Don't forget to make a follow-up appointment with the OB who delivered your baby. Make the appointment within four to six weeks after the delivery (that means you'll have to call for an appointment as soon as you get home—you know how these doctors are with their schedules). If you have any questions regarding your recovery, however, always call your doctor ASAP.

As far as wound care goes, you can take a shower, but don't rub the incision while showering. Let the water run over it and take a bar of antibacterial soap, make a dollop of suds in your hands and apply it gently to the incision, let the suds sit for a minute, and then rinse them off. Use a clean towel and pat the incision dry, don't rub it. If you want to use Bacitracin or Neosporin ointment and rub it on, it might reduce scarring. (But, first make sure you're not allergic to either of those products.) Taking a bath is acceptable once your bleeding has decreased significantly. Be careful not to slip while getting out of the tub. For the first couple of weeks, a shower is preferable.

note

In case you're wondering about what effects the medications may have on the baby, don't be overly concerned. A small amount of the medications will appear in the breast milk; however, this has not been shown to have a detrimental effect on the baby. In addition, the mother probably won't be taking these medications long enough to potentially harm the baby.

For painkillers, the majority of women can take Motrin or Ibuprofen. Make sure you take any medicine with food or milk, assuming that there are no contraindications to that. Take medicine regularly for the first couple of days after surgery. Most doctors will also provide a narcotic-based medicine as well. Dr. John recommends trying the Ibuprofen first and then the narcotics—the reason being, Ibuprofen is an anti-inflammatory, which will address the cause of the problem, whereas the narcotic simply masks the pain. Be aware that the Ibuprofen might have gastro-intestinal side effects. The narcotics also have side effects, including drowsiness, which could increase your chances for clotting and constipation if you're sleeping and not walking (unless, of course, you sleepwalk). Instead, try taking the narcotic at night if you're going to take it.

For the six weeks after surgery, use walking as your main source of exercise. Avoid setups or crunches or anything that could weaken or tear the incision.

The Unexpected C-Section

Obviously, if you have an unexpected c-section, then it is probably an emergency situation. Many of the same procedures will be followed, but probably faster—OK, possibly at lightning or warp speed on the part of the hospital staff. The father or significant other may or may not be allowed in the operating room. It will depend on the severity of the situation.

The Absolute Minimum

There is no getting around the fact that a c-section is an operation that requires cutting, and as such, it can be dangerous. Fortunately, with the advent of antibiotics and improvements in surgical techniques, it is a relatively normal procedure that is performed routinely and successfully every day around the world. Still, be aware of what it entails and ask questions before you get to the point where you need a c-section.

- If you can avoid a c-section, do so. Vaginal deliveries are always preferable in terms of safety, unless there is a medical contraindication.
- Most c-sections are safe, and you shouldn't worry too much about the outcome for you or your baby.
- Follow your doctor's advice carefully both pre-op and post-op. Your wellness depends on your attention to detail.
- Make sure you have plenty of help after the baby is born. You will be sore for quite a while and will need some help getting around.

IN THIS CHAPTER

- Who takes care of the baby once it is born?
- How does the Apgar test work?
- Signs and symptoms of jaundice in an infant
- Statewide screening tests for babies and how they work

18

WHAT HAPPENS TO THE BABY AFTER DELIVERY?

This chapter title seems like a question with an obvious answer. Your first reaction is probably well, duh…the baby is hugged, loved, kissed, and welcomed to this world. But not all babies who are born are healthy and ready to be greeted in quite this fashion. And whether or not you realize it, there is a medical team present and ready to help your baby, if necessary, when it is born.

Houston, We Have a Baby!

Shortly after the baby's birth, whether it's a vaginal birth or a c-section, the baby will be evaluated for its ability to adapt and transition normally to life outside the uterus. To aid in this process, the baby is transported to a warming unit with a radiant heat source. The baby (now officially called a *neonate*) is dried of all moisture, which helps to minimize the loss of its core temperature.

The nose and mouth of the baby are suctioned to clear the baby of all secretions and to aid in its first breathing efforts. The baby should begin crying within the first 30 seconds to one minute of life. To accomplish this, gentle stimulation is usually required and accomplished by rubbing the baby's back or gently stimulating its feet.

DANGLING BABIES

Some of you may be familiar with old movies or books that described or depicted the delivering physician as holding up the baby by its feet in mid air and spanking the baby's bottom (translation: bare butt) in order to get the baby to cry. This procedure is no longer done because it isn't necessary. According to Dr. John, it was an accepted practice because doctors simply didn't know any better, and they went overboard a tad. Today's doctors know that aggressive stimulation isn't necessary, and it could potentially harm the baby. For example, the baby could be dropped or hit too hard in a vulnerable spot that might injure it.

The Neonatal Team Takes Over

Usually, when the delivery is approaching, the patient's nurse will call for additional personnel to manage the baby's transition. These individuals are referred to as NRPs (neonatal resuscitative providers). They may be doctors, nurses, or medical assistants, but all of them have special training in the initial evaluation of and resuscitation of newborns.

And the Ranking Is...Enter the Apgar Score

The baby's attendants will begin their initial evaluation at one and five minutes after birth, using the Apgar scoring system. The intent of the Apgar score is to provide a quick evaluation of a newborn and determine if additional measures of resuscitation are necessary. Apgar scores range from zero to 10. In general, a low Apgar identifies those babies who may require extra attention and care. The five-minute Apgar score is generally used to evaluate how effective any resuscitative efforts were.

The Apgar table is comprised of five areas in which the baby will receive a score. These areas include the baby's heart rate, muscle tone, respiratory effort, reflexive response to stimulation, and the baby's color (see Table 18.1).

Table 18.1 The APGAR Scoring System

Sign	0	1	2
Heart Rate	Absent	< 100 per minute	> 100 per minute
Respiratory Effort	Apneic	Weak, Irregular, Gasping	Regular
Reflex	No Response	Some Response	Facial Grimace, Sneeze, Cough
Muscle Tone	Flaccid	Some Flexion	Good Flexion of Arms and Legs
Color	Blue, Pale	Body Pink, Hands and Feet Blue	Pink

A value of 0, 1, or 2 is assigned to each category, and this gives the baby its overall score out of 10. Generally, Apgar scores in the range of 7–10 suggest that the baby doesn't require additional resuscitative efforts; however, a score between 4–7 is considered an indicator that the baby may be mildly to moderately compromised (needing attention). In those babies with a score less than 4, the rating usually indicates that the baby might need oxygen and additional attention from the medical staff. (According to Dr. John, medical people joke around and say that no babies ever get a perfect 10, unless they are a pediatrician's baby.)

MY PERFECT "10"

The birth of my third child (and first daughter) was something of a fiasco of my own making. I was at a teaching hospital, but didn't realize what that meant when they asked me if I'd mind having a "few" nurses observe the delivery. When they wheeled me into an amphitheater-type room, it was too late to protest. OK, 15 nurses (some male—I'd forgotten there was such a thing as male nurses) gathered round to watch under spotlights. So much for intimate, personal deliveries with the lights dimmed. If I hadn't been so preoccupied having a baby, I would have been mortified.

The only good part was that they clapped when I delivered, and my daughter was a perfect "10" on the Apgar scale—at 1 minute and at 5 minutes. (I think it had something to do with the movie "10" being popular several years earlier.) In retrospect, it was the only way for my drama-queen daughter to make her appearance onto the stage of life.

The Nursery

If the baby is doing well and is considered stable, then it can spend a short time with its mother before proceeding to the nursery. At the nursery the baby will be cleaned more thoroughly, as well as evaluated once again.

Immediately after the baby is born, it becomes the patient of another doctor (not your OB, but one who is expert in the care of newborns). The general evaluation of a normal newborn includes the observation of the baby's transition from intrauterine to extra uterine life. The neonatal teams will be establishing feeding habits of either the breast or the bottle, watching for normal patterns of urination and bowel movements, and keeping an overall surveillance of the baby for any problems. Concerning signs might include a change in the baby's activity rate, a refusal to eat, temperature changes, skin color changes, jaundice, a rapid respiratory rate, or vomiting. The neonatal team will also be giving vaccinations if necessary and doing mandatory state screening tests on the infant.

tip

Don't forget to interview and line up a pediatrician or a general practice physician *before* you go to the hospital to have your baby. You need to make sure that there is a physician ready to care for your baby the minute it is born, just in case.

What Is Jaundice?

The most common difficulty in newborns is jaundice (yellow-looking skin), and in most cases it will disappear in two weeks or less without any special treatment. For most full-term babies, jaundice should not last longer than one week.

Jaundice occurs when excess bilirubin is released into the baby's circulation, caused by the destruction of circulating red blood cells. Jaundice may be attributed to physiological causes (immaturity of the baby's liver), prematurity, breast milk (occuring in one to two percent of breastfed babies), blood group incompatibility (Rh or ABO problems), or hepatitis (rare).

If a doctor does a blood test and decides to treat the baby, the baby will be placed under special lights (also known as *phototherapy*). If jaundice is prolonged or associated with other metabolic abnormalities, additional measures may be necessary.

A small percentage of babies who are breast-fed can develop breast milk jaundice. The cause of this is not entirely clear, but it's thought to be related to the composition of the mother's milk. It's normal for breast-fed babies to have higher bilirubin levels than formula-fed babies; however, the mother should continue to breast-feed.

The nursery will weigh the baby for the first time. Contrary to popular belief, the baby is not weighed right after delivery for a couple of reasons. First, there is no baby scale in the delivery room. Second, the neonatal providers have more important responsibilities when taking care of the baby than determining its weight. Although the weight is important and the most common question that parents ask, the baby will be weighed and measured later at the nursery's convenience.

The baby will be wrapped snugly in a baby blanket and placed under the warmer whenever it's not with the mother. The mother provides warmth to the baby by holding it close and transferring her own heat to it. When the mother is not holding the baby, she's asked to keep the baby wrapped in a blanket to aid in heat preservation. When the baby is cold, extra energy is expended to maintain its core temperature, and this can add stress to the baby if it occurs for a prolonged period of time.

If the baby is showing any signs of distress, which could be caused by an infection or a metabolic disorder, the baby may undergo blood tests. Amazingly, there are tiny blood pressure cuffs that can be placed around the baby's arms or legs to measure blood pressure. If necessary, intravenous lines may be placed in the baby so that it can receive extra fluids and medicines. However, most babies don't require these measures or anything much beyond the initial evaluation. The more reassuring and healthy the baby appears to the nursery staff, the sooner the baby will be returned to the mother for bonding.

If the mother desires, she can begin breast-feeding shortly after the birth, but the baby may be tired and want to sleep for several hours before its first feeding. And it goes without saying that the mother may be tired as well.

Shortly after the baby's birth, the hospital will notify your pediatrician, and he or she will visit the hospital to check on the baby's status. At that time, the pediatrician will probably perform some of his or her own tests. The nursery will also give the baby a series of immunizations, one of which is the hepatitis vaccine.

SPOTTING JAUNDICE IN YOUR BABY

Jaundice usually begins around the second to third day of life. The baby's face will appear yellow first and then the color will spread to its chest and legs. The whites of the eyes can also be yellow.

To test for jaundice, press your fingertip on the tip of your child's nose or forehead. If the skin shows white (works for all races), then there is no jaundice. If the skin is yellow or slightly yellow, contact your pediatrician immediately. Because many babies are released from the hospital before the baby develops jaundice, it is up to the parents to spot it. Remember: jaundice can be dangerous to the baby, possibly causing deafness, cerebral palsy, brain damage, or even indicating the presence of hepatitis.

Screening Tests for Newborns

Each newborn baby gets its heel pricked for a blood test, but the specific tests that blood gets screened for depends on the state where you live.

There are several rare conditions that can be picked up in a screening and save lives (for example, some genetic diseases and immune disorders). Find out what your state screens for and make the decision yourself whether or not you want to pay for additional screening if it's not offered. Usually, you can order a test from a private laboratory that may be fairly inexpensive (it may cost as little as an extra $25), and that test can give you peace of mind if it is negative, or save a life if it is positive.

> **tip**
>
> Check your state's Web site or call your state health department for more information on the tests your state requires. If you can't get the information there, be proactive and ask your hospital ahead of time.

THE ABSOLUTE MINIMUM

Finally, finally, finally, you have a baby! Rest up while you're still in the hospital and enjoy that wonderful new being in your life. But that new infant brings with it a new set of mind-boggling responsibilities. You will immediately be thrust into parenthood, and it starts right now.

- Once the baby is born, you'll have a chance to connect with him (or her) for a few minutes—and longer if the baby is healthy.
- Suddenly, you'll realize that there are additional people in the delivery room, and the extra ones are devoted to taking care of your new baby (what a relief!).
- Choose a pediatrician (or general practitioner for the baby) ahead of time so that your baby is in good hands once it is born.
- Be an aware parent—know what to look for in case your baby develops jaundice. Also, decide in advance what types of screening tests you want your baby to have, regardless of what the state offers. Make sure that you know what vaccinations are suggested or required for a newborn.

IN THIS CHAPTER

- What feelings are normal?
- The difference between the "blues" and depression
- Coping mechanisms and skills vs. meds
- Medicine as opposed to herbal remedies
- When to get help
- What is serious depression?

19

POSTPARTUM BLUES AND POSTPARTUM DEPRESSION

We've all heard about postpartum depression and the "baby blues," which have been in the forefront of the news recently due to some deaths that were attributed to one mother's postpartum depression. The court case highlights the fact that even experts disagree as to how and why postpartum depression occurs. Is it a valid defense? We'll leave that up to the courts. In this chapter, we'll try to differentiate between temporary hormonal depression (the "blues") and more serious postpartum depression or psychosis, giving you some ways to cope and deal with emotional issues and the physical changes you might experience.

There are three classifications of postpartum depression (known as PPD in the medical profession):

- Postpartum blues
- Postpartum depression
- Postpartum psychosis

Postpartum Blues

It's perfectly normal to experience the postpartum "blues" (sometimes referred to as the "baby blues"), which mothers usually notice shortly after delivery ("shortly" being defined as within two hours to two weeks after delivery). This condition occurs in over half of all new mothers, and it is thought to be caused by hormonal changes.

Symptoms

Symptoms of postpartum blues may include the following:

- Sleep disturbances
- Difficulty with concentration
- Sudden mood swings (very happy to very sad)
- Frequent crying
- Irritability or impatience
- Loneliness or sadness/depression

tip

Not everyone experiences postpartum blues, so if you don't get them, consider yourself fortunate. Some women only experience the blues for a few hours. I was one of the fortunate ones. I was always so ecstatic not to be pregnant any longer that nothing could have marred my joy!

Postpartum blues usually go away on their own within two weeks of having the baby, so there is often no need to take medications for the condition. As the body returns to normal, the depression disappears.

Doctors like to prepare their patients for the possibility of postpartum depression, so that women are educated in advance and understand what is happening. They also try to prepare the husband and family so that they will understand the difference between normal blues and true postpartum depression.

FATHERS GET THE BLUES, TOO

Women aren't the only ones affected by depression. New fathers can also experience symptoms of depression. For a lot of guys, having a baby can be a mixed blessing. Although they may be proud and pleased to have offspring, they can also be torn by the emotional and financial obligations of fatherhood—not to mention their changed social strata. Hey, it's a huge change in lifestyle when you have to have a babysitter in order to leave the house!

Men also might feel left out when the new baby arrives or feel torn about sharing their wife with a baby (or even envious of the partnership that the mother and baby seem to have). Be sensitive to your partner's needs. Include him and make his relationship with the baby as important as yours—it is, after all. Also be aware that your partner might need some counseling or just to talk to someone (perhaps his own father or an older man).

Dealing with the Blues

In general, it is wise to be kind to yourself during this period, particularly if it's your first baby. Having a baby is a major life experience that involves a wide range of emotions from being deliriously happy at one moment to panicked and afraid the next moment. All of these feelings are normal. Family and friends should reassure you and take away some of the pressure, if possible. If you don't have a good support system in place, there are always community service organizations available with counselors. Use them for help of any kind—that's why they are there.

The blues can occur for any number of good reasons (besides the obvious hormonal ones). You may be worried about being a good mother, have financial concerns, wonder about the baby's health, or any of the other normal headaches of daily life that occur when you have a baby. For example, what do you do when the baby cries? Are you getting enough sleep? Is the baby sleeping and eating properly? Will you have enough money to support this child? Will your husband be a good father? Or will the baby be OK without a father if you're not married?

All of these questions are valid, and you're justified in worrying about them, but try to put off focusing on them for a few weeks after your baby is born. Instead, breathe deeply, think calm thoughts, get plenty of rest, take walks, and in general, take good care of yourself. You are the baby's most important person. Let yourself enjoy your baby and your new life.

Also, think about joining a support group for new mothers (or form one of your own). Check with your hospital to see if they offer any programs. Simply talking to other mothers will help you realize that you're not alone. Other mothers should be able to answer some of your questions. There are also a number of good Web sites online that can answer any questions, and Web sites are a good alternative if you're hesitant to leave your baby to attend support meetings.

tip

If at all possible, the best advice is to plan for some of these situations before the baby is born, so that your concerns will be alleviated or at least addressed in advance of the baby's birth.

GETTING HELP ONLINE

I can't personally recommend any of these sites, but when I did a Google search on the words "Pregnancy Chat Rooms," these were some of the sites that came up:

- `www.ivillage.com`
- `www.groups.msn.com/SinglePregnant/Women/messageboard.msnw`
- `www.globalwomensnet.com/pregnancy/pregnancyforums`

I visited one or two of them, and the women seemed to be open about discussing their lives and supporting one another. Here is an example taken directly (and unedited) from a site for single expectant mothers.

One woman wrote:

"Hi. I am 29 and am 24 weeks pregnant. The father left me after 4 years to date a 21-year-old. He wants nothing to do with myself (sic) nor our daughter who will be here shortly. How do I stop crying? He wanted an abortion, I said no. I know in the end he will be missing out, but right now I feel I am the only one suffering...."

Another woman's response:

"You are not the only one suffering! We are all suffering along with you...you are NOT alone in this. I'm 32, 14 weeks preg and my boyfriend who promised to marry me is leaving me. I have days where I feel so sad, then days when I am excited about beginning a new life. Just get through these bad days, a good day is right around the corner. Trust in your friends and family they love you and want to help. My parents are both deceased and I only have 2 brothers for family left (no Aunts or Uncles). I never used to talk to my brothers, but they are doing all they can to help me through with this now. Believe me, there are people out there you mean the world to and once your daughter is born, she'll be your biggest fan. :-)"

Online help is not the answer to depression, but it could help you feel more connected to other women and to know that you're not alone.

Postpartum Depression

Postpartum depression (PPD) is more serious than the blues, and it may occur a few days after childbirth or as late as a few months after the birth.

Symptoms

The feelings of postpartum depression mimic the feelings experienced with the blues and might include all or some of the following symptoms:

- Depression
- Anxiety
- Loneliness
- Irritability
- Despair
- Lack of energy
- Overeating and weight gain
- Inability to eat or weight loss
- Overly worried about the baby
- Sleeplessness or sleeping too much
- Feeling guilty or worthless
- No interest in fun activities, pleasure, or sex
- No interest in the baby
- Being afraid of hurting yourself or the baby

The Difference Between Postpartum Blues and Postpartum Depression

The major difference between postpartum blues and postpartum depression is the severity with which you experience these feelings (see Figure 19.1). In postpartum depression, you have these feelings more strongly than the blues. Rather than just feeling occasional sadness, the sad feelings become overwhelming and seem to control your life. Postpartum depression can start soon after birth or even begin during the pregnancy (which obviously makes us wonder why they lump it in with postpartum). Or it can happen anytime during the first year after the baby's birth, which is a fact that most women don't realize. However, if it's going to happen, it usually peaks at about two to four months after the baby is born.

If you are experiencing depression that lasts more than two weeks, and you have any of the symptoms listed above, then you should be tested for PPD by your healthcare provider. Women in this condition are often unable to take care of themselves or their babies.

tip

If postpartum blues occur in half of all women, postpartum depression happens in less than 15 percent of the population. It is a much less common occurrence.

How to Treat PPD

PPD can be treated in a number of ways. The first and least invasive way is to visit a therapist. Often, just talking through the issues will be enough to get you over the hump and feeling better. A therapist can give you clarity about the issues you're facing and suggest different ways of handling them, rather than bottling them up. You can find a therapist in the phone book or get a recommendation from your doctor or friends. Or, if you can't afford a therapist, try talking to a close friend or relative, a clergy person, a healthcare worker, or a social worker—anyone whom you trust and whose opinion you value.

Although there are many herbal remedies for depression (St. John's Wert, etc.), doctors don't usually recommend them before conventional medicine. The conventional drugs have been rigorously studied and tested, and the drug companies have a vested interest in making sure the medicine does what it says it will. On the other hand, over-the-counter herbal remedies don't have to submit to the rigorous testing and requirements of the FDA (Food and Drug Administration). You can't always be sure what you're taking.

note

As far as specific antidepressants go, Prozac, Paxil, Zoloft and other medicines of this type (SSRIs) are generally safe to take, and so far there is no known association between these meds and congenital anomalies.

And don't forget the basics: Eating right, getting as much rest as possible, and exercising are all natural and effective ways of dealing with less-serious depression (and they can't hurt you).

Can I Breastfeed if I'm on an Anti-Depressant Medication?

As far as breastfeeding is concerned, it's unclear if anti-depressant medication poses any risks to the baby. In most cases, it's OK to nurse, but all women need to know that anti-depressants are secreted in the breast milk, meaning the baby will be exposed to them as the baby nurses. In general, most doctors feel the risk is worth taking if the mother needs the medication, since there are so many good things to be gained from nursing (in other words, risks offset benefits).

However, there are some ways to lessen the effects of the medications (if your doctor agrees). If the baby is on a feeding schedule, then you can feed the baby when the drug is at its lowest level in the mother's body. For example, if you are taking meds four times a day (every six hours), then you can try to breastfeed around the fifth hour when the medicine is at its lowest level. Of course, this should be discussed first with both your OB and your pediatrician.

caution

Women who have been on anti-depressants throughout their pregnancy may find that their baby exhibits signs of withdrawal when the baby is born. For example, the baby may be jittery or have problems feeding. Doctors are constantly re-evaluating patients on anti-depressants. The criteria for giving a prescription is a balancing act. Physicians would prefer *not* to have women on any drugs, but they understand the small but potential risks are sometimes worth taking.

It's also a good idea to let your obstetrician and pediatrician know what your psychiatrist is recommending and vice versa, so that all your doctors are aware of your needs and progress and can coordinate their prescriptions.

POSTPARTUM ANXIETY

Yet another disorder that could occur, but is more rare, is called *postpartum* anxiety or panic disorder. The signs of this disorder mimic normal panic disorder and include strong anxiety or fear, rapid breathing, a fast heart rate, hot or cold flashes, feeling disoriented or shaky or dizzy, and possibly experiencing chest pain. If you have any of these symptoms, talk to your doctor immediately. Medication and counseling can treat this disorder.

caution

Do not breastfeed if you are taking Lithium, which is commonly used to treat bipolar disorder, because there is a risk of Lithium toxicity to the baby. Also avoid amphetamines, which can be dangerous for the baby.

Postpartum Psychosis

The third tier of depression, which represents the worst of the PPDs, is postpartum psychosis. This is the most serious of the postpartum disorders, but fortunately, it's very rare and only occurs in one to two women per thousand deliveries. Like the other types of depression, it can happen as early as a few hours or days after the baby is born.

Symptoms

Symptoms of postpartum psychosis can include all or part of the following:

- Anxiety
- Confusion
- Agitation
- Restless
- Sleeplessness
- Hallucinations
- Delusional thoughts about yourself or the baby
- Thoughts about harming yourself or the baby (elevated risk of suicide or homicide)

This type of depression usually occurs in someone who has a history of depression herself or a genetic family history of depression. Other risk factors include someone who doesn't have support mechanisms in place, had something traumatic happen during the pregnancy, or has a previous history of bipolar disorder or some other psychotic disorder.

caution

Women who have a history of depression occurring in a pregnancy, will have a 50 percent chance of recurrence in their next pregnancy.

Treatment

In almost all cases of postpartum psychosis, the patient is hospitalized immediately and treated with some kind of medication and counseling. The prognosis for mother and baby is good if the mother seeks help.

FROM THE DOCTOR'S PERSPECTIVE...

When Dr. John was stationed in Italy, one of his patients was the wife of a Navy enlisted man. "She looked fairly normal during pregnancy, although there were some control issues on the part of her husband," said Dr. John and continued. "I remember that the woman was fairly passive during her pregnancy while her husband was talking. When I asked her about problems at home and depression (as doctors, we always ask), she never admitted to anything, such as anxiety or sleep issues. However, on the second postpartum day, she was very depressed and agitated, which was uncharacteristic for her when I was following her prenatally. She admitted to me that she thought she might hurt herself or the baby. I had psychiatric services meet with her and a social worker as well. I also notified child protective services so that they would check in with her when she got home. I placed her on antidepressants, and she felt better within four to six months. Looking back, I think she probably had had depression before the pregnancy or during it, or she might even have had a personality disorder or other psychiatric condition."

The Absolute Minimum

The most important thing to remember about any kind of depression is to seek help from the medical community ASAP. If your doctor doesn't seem to be worried or listening to you, then find someone else who will.

- Most women experience some depression after the birth of their baby. This is normal and will pass in time.
- If you're experiencing mild depression, do your part to get rid of it. Eat well, get plenty of sleep (have other people assist you with the baby), and exercise. Talk to your spouse or friends about your fears or concerns. Try to alleviate any exacerbating situations that make you feel worse.
- Get counseling if at all possible.
- Depression can be a dangerous thing for all concerned. If you notice symptoms in yourself, act on them. If your doctor doesn't take you seriously, find another doctor who will listen to you.

Glossary

American College of Obstetrics and Gynecology ACOG is a nonprofit member organization comprised of physicians dedicated to the advancement of women's health.

amniocentesis A diagnostic procedure where a small amount of amniotic fluid that surrounds the baby is removed and tested for the presence of a genetic disorder, fetal abnormality, or infection.

amniotic fluid The fluid contained by the amniotic sac that surrounds and supports the fetus during pregnancy.

anesthesiologist In pregnancy, the physician who specializes in pain management during labor and delivery and also handles the administration of epidurals and general anesthesia.

Apgar test The Apgar test is comprised of five components in which the baby receives a score after birth. The point of the test is to do a quick evaluation of the baby's health at one and five minutes after birth.

bikini cut Typically called a *Pfannenstiel skin incision*, this is a horizontal incision just above the pubic hairline, ergo the bikini line. It is associated with c-sections.

Braxton Hicks contractions These are irregular contractions (tightening of the uterus) that are called *false* because they aren't associated with true labor—that is, the cervix doesn't dilate with these contractions. (They can feel real, though.)

CBC (complete blood count) A blood test that checks your hematocrit and hemoglobin, as well as platelet count (in other words, measures your potential for anemia and the ability to clot). It is usually one of the first tests performed after you find out you're pregnant.

Certified Nurse Midwives (CNMs) A nurse who has completed additional training and certification to manage uncomplicated pregnancies, as well as labor and delivery.

cervix A portion of the uterus that undergoes changes during labor that allows the baby to pass through the birth canal. Normally, it is closed until labor begins.

cesarean section (more commonly referred to as a **c-section**) In a c-section the baby does not travel through the birth canal, but instead is pulled out through an incision made in the mother's abdomen and uterus. It is performed in an operating room under sterile conditions, and is considered to be major surgery.

chlamydia A bacteria that is commonly associated with infections of the female genital tract and is responsible for infections of the baby. It can cause pre-term labor.

circumcision The removal of a baby boy's foreskin by cutting it.

classical c-section In this type of c-section, the physician makes an incision or cut in the upper portion of the uterus. The advantage is that it gives more access to the baby. The disadvantage is that it leaves a larger scar on the mother and makes subsequent vaginal deliveries difficult to impossible.

contraction A tightening of the uterus that causes labor to progress. They are regular in duration and interval spacing, which means, for example, that they might occur every two minutes and last for 30 seconds each.

dilatation Process by which the cervix expands. During labor, it is measured in centimeters.

Doppler monitor A fetal heart monitor that is attached to the mother's abdomen during labor to track the baby's heart rate.

dysfunctional labor pattern This condition occurs when labor is slow to progress or stops for some reason.

effacement Describes the thinning of the cervix during labor. Commonly measured in percentages during a cervical exam.

episiotomy A process by which a doctor makes an incision or cut in the space between the vagina and rectum in order to expand the opening for the baby's head.

false contractions *See Braxton Hicks contractions.*

false negative This result from a pregnancy test indicates that you are not pregnant, when in fact, you are pregnant. The test is in error.

false positive This result from a pregnancy test indicates that you are pregnant, when in fact, you are not pregnant. The test is in error.

family practitioner A physician who specializes in primary care medicine and who also manages uncomplicated pregnancies, as well as labor and delivery.

fetal alcohol syndrome An adverse outcome affecting the baby; it is caused by excessive maternal consumption of alcohol during pregnancy.

fetus The developing pregnancy in the uterus near the end of the first trimester until birth.

first stage of labor This stage occurs at the beginning of labor when you are having regular contractions with cervical change, i.e., you are in labor.

first trimester This is the first three months of your pregnancy (weeks 1–12).

FMLA (Family and Medical Leave Act of 1993) Federal legislation that entitles most employees to take a total of up to 12 weeks of unpaid leave from their job following the birth of a baby.

forceps A medical instrument that looks like overly large tongs and is used to pull out the baby through the vagina.

GBS (group B streptococcus) A bacterial strain present in 20–25% of women. It poses no threat to the mother, but can be lethal for the baby.

gestational diabetes A diabetic condition in pregnant women that is caused by the pregnancy. It usually subsides after the birth of the baby.

glucose tolerance test A blood test that is performed at the end of the second trimester which screens for the presence of gestational diabetes.

gonorrhea A sexually transmitted disease in the mother that can contribute to complications of the mother and newborn.

hepatitis B A virus transmitted by infusion of infected blood or through needles or via sexual intercourse; it causes inflammation of the liver. Hepatitis B can be transmitted to the baby during delivery or through breast-feeding, and it also can cause pre-term labor.

HIV The human immunodeficiency virus. A sexually transmitted virus that can be contracted through blood products or shared needles, and it also can cause AIDS. It has a high transmission rate to babies in untreated mothers.

hyperplasia The increase in the number of cells in the baby. Occurs primarily in the first trimester.

hypertrophy The growth of cells that have already formed. Generally occurs after the first trimester and lasts throughout the rest of the pregnancy.

Isoimmunization The development of antibodies to red blood cell markers following exposure to such markers from another individual. In pregnancy, the other individual is the fetus.

IUPC (intrauterine pressure catheter) A flexible probe inserted through the vagina that occupies the space between the baby and the interior uterine wall to detect the strength, frequency, and durations of contractions.

jaundice Jaundice occurs when excess bilirubin is released into the baby's circulation, which is caused by the destruction of circulating red blood cells. The baby's skin looks yellowish in color when it is jaundiced.

Kegel exercises Exercises to strengthen the muscle group (the *pubococcygeous muscle or pc muscle)* that aids in controlling the flow of urine.

kick counts Also known as *fetal kick counts,* this is a procedure a mother can perform at home in order to assess the baby's well-being. The actual kick count is determined by counting the baby's kicks over a certain time period.

low-transverse c-section (LTCS) In a low-transverse c-section, the doctor cuts through the lower uterine segment of the uterus. The advantage of this surgery is that a woman could potentially deliver her next baby by the vaginal route with a lower risk of the uterus rupturing, compared to a classical c-section.

midwife *See CNMs.*

miscarriage The unintended loss of a pregnancy usually within the first trimester.

mucous plug The substance that occupies the cervical canal; it dislodges during the early stages of labor. It is usually pink in color, secondary to a small amount of bloodstaining.

multiple marker screen A blood test usually performed during the second trimester. This test screens for the various genetic disorders, as well as spina bifida.

Naegele's Rule A way to calculate your delivery date. Take the first day of your last menstrual period, subtract three months, add seven days, and that should be your due date (usually 40 weeks).

neonatal care The part of the hospital that takes care of newborn babies.

NICU (neonatal intensive care unit) Usually a Level III nursery where babies who are very sick receive special care and monitoring after birth.

obstetrician/gynecologist (OB/GYN) A physician who specializes in women's health care; this includes management of complicated and uncomplicated pregnancies, as well as labor and delivery.

pap smear A test designed to screen for cervical cancer.

Pfannenstiel skin incision *See bikini cut.*

pitocin A medicine that stimulates the uterine to contract. Often given to help induce or augment labor.

placenta The organ by which the fetus obtains its nourishment through the umbilical cord.

placenta previa Occurs when the placenta implants over or very near the internal opening of the cervix. This can be a source of profuse bleeding, often occurring in the third trimester. It usually necessitates a c-section delivery.

postpartum The period of time after the baby is delivered in which the mother recovers from the effects of labor and delivery and the pregnancy.

postpartum blues A period of time shortly after birth when the mother feels sad or depressed (a feeling of being letdown). This common condition can occur within two hours to two weeks after the baby is born. Also called the *baby blues.*

postpartum depression A more serious form of depression after the birth of a baby. It is differentiated from the blues by the fact that it doesn't go away and is more severe.

postpartum psychosis This is the worst form of depression associated with pregnancy and often requires hospitalization. It usually occurs in someone who has a history of depression. Get help for this condition immediately!

pre-eclampsia A unique and serious form of hypertension or high blood pressure associated with protein in the urine that occurs during pregnancy. The only known cure today is the birth of the baby.

pre-term labor This condition occurs when the mother goes into labor in advance of her normal due date (usually the baby is less than 36 weeks gestation). Pre-term labor can be dangerous for both the mother and the baby.

prolapsed cord This condition refers to the umbilical cord coming out in advance of the baby's head. It is an emergency situation due to the fact that the circulation to the baby could be cut off by compression of the cord.

RhoGAM An immunoglobulin medicine that is prescribed for women who are RH negative, usually taken at 28 weeks of pregnancy and within 72 hours of delivery. This helps to prevent isoimmunization *(see also isoimmunization).*

rubella screen This screen tests for the presence of the virus rubella, which is capable of causing fetal abnormalities from a maternal infection during the first trimester of pregnancy. It's also called *German measles*.

second stage of labor The second stage of labor occurs when the cervix is maximally dilated (10 centimeters); at this point, the mother is told she can push.

second trimester This is the time period between 13 and 27 weeks of your pregnancy.

syphilis screen This screen tests for the presence of syphilis, which is a sexually transmitted disease that can cause preterm labor, death of the baby, or congenital anomalies.

third stage of labor This stage begins after the baby has been delivered and lasts until the placenta comes out (usually less than 30 minutes).

third trimester This is the time period between 28 weeks to the end of the pregnancy (delivery).

ultrasound A medical device that uses sound waves; it is often used to evaluate the baby's condition and measure the amount of amniotic fluid.

umbilical cord The cord that connects the placenta to the baby and allows the transfer of nutrients and waste products between the baby and mother.

uterine contraction monitor A device in the labor and delivery room that is hooked up to the mother to monitor her contractions.

UTI (urinary tract infection) This infection is picked up by a urine screen. Pregnant women are more prone to UTIs during pregnancy than they are normally.

vacuum A device usually made of plastic that is placed over the baby's head that can aid in the delivery of the baby. It creates suction to pull the baby out through the vagina.

Western blot analysis Women who test positive for AIDS on their initial screening will be given this test. If the tests are positive, then a diagnosis of HIV infection is made and medications can be given to reduce the risk of transmission to the baby.

Index

A

B

How can we make this index more useful? Email us at indexes@quepublishing.com

F

G

H

I

J-K

L

M

N

O

P

Q-R

S

T

U

How can we make this index more useful? Email us at indexes@quepublishing.com

V

W-Z